Dermatological Manual of Outdoor Hazards

Julian Trevino · Amy Y-Y Chen
Editors

Dermatological Manual of Outdoor Hazards

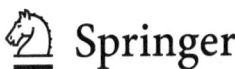 Springer

Editors
Julian Trevino
Boonshoft School of Medicine
Wright State University
Dayton, OH, USA

Amy Y-Y Chen
Central Connecticut Dermatology
Cromwell, CT, USA

ISBN 978-3-030-37781-6   ISBN 978-3-030-37782-3   (eBook)
https://doi.org/10.1007/978-3-030-37782-3

This Springer imprint is published by the registered company Springer Nature Switzerland AG
The registered company address is: Gewerbestrasse 11, 6330 Cham, Switzerland

Preface

Hazardous exposures to arthropods and plants involve millions of patients annually and are becoming more frequent due to an ever-expanding array of outdoor occupational and recreational activities and increased domestic and international travel. Such exposures can result in skin conditions and systemic manifestations which range from minor annoyances to life-threatening illnesses. Arthropod vectors transmit diseases affecting millions and resulting in significant public health issues worldwide. Exposures to plants can affect exposed populations and result in significant morbidity (and rarely mortality), necessitating alteration in occupational/recreational activities or requiring limitations in dietary consumption of implicated plants. Media reports of exaggerated information on the adverse effects of plant and arthropod exposures abound. Physicians and healthcare providers in a variety of practice settings are in a unique position to provide accurate information about such exposures as well as to diagnose and manage adverse reactions to plants and arthropods. It is hoped that this manual will be utilized as a trusted reference for those seeking information on accurately diagnosing and managing such hazardous plant and arthropod exposures.

This manual provides an organized approach to recognition, diagnosis, and management of hazardous exposure to plants and arthropods. Following a review of skin lesion morphology and terminology, the subsequent chapters review the broad range of skin manifestations due to plant exposures based on the underlying pathogenic mechanism (plant-induced urticaria, irritant plant dermatitis, allergic contact dermatitis, phytophotodermatitis). The full spectrum of plant-induced dermatitis, emphasizing routes of exposure, plant identification, and clues to arriving at a diagnosis and providing effective management and preventative strategies, is presented. The remainder of the manual reviews the broad array of skin manifestations and related systemic findings due to exposure to a wide variety of arthropods. Due to their individual bites/stings and their role as vectors of disease worldwide, arthropod injuries to the skin and the systemic diseases resulting from some arthropod exposures can present significant diagnostic and therapeutic challenges to clinicians. The chapters on arthropod exposures will provide guidance to healthcare professional in the diagnosis, management, and prevention of such exposures.

Throughout the manual, emphasis is placed on obtaining pertinent historical information (e.g., exposure through occupational or recreational activities, pet/animal exposure, clothing worn, fragrances used, travel history), recognition of characteristic clinical findings, and appropriate patient evaluation and management. Preventative measures (use of repellants, protective clothing, barrier creams) and patient education are also emphasized as relate to the various exposures. While clinical manifestations of the various exposures can range from non-specific to highly characteristic, the manual provides a framework for healthcare professionals to comprehensively assess suspected plant and arthropod exposures and ultimately arrive at an accurate diagnosis.

Depending on practice location, physicians and providers may see some of these conditions infrequently and thus a review and update on this information is essential. With increasing mobility of populations and the ease of worldwide travel, a condition normally seen thousands of miles away can now suddenly present to a practitioner anywhere on the planet for evaluation. Physicians/providers should be familiar with potentially serious medical consequences and infectious conditions/complications related to cutaneous reactions resulting from specific plants and arthropods in order to deliver a rapid diagnosis, effective treatment, and comprehensive education to patients regarding safe and effective measures for management and prevention of hazardous plant and arthropod exposures. This manual will serve as a trusted resource to clinicians seeking to deliver outstanding care to such patients.

Dayton, USA   Julian Trevino M.D.
Cromwell, USA   Amy Y-Y Chen M.D.

Acknowledgements

This manual represents the efforts of a team of gifted individuals. Sincere thanks to all of the contributing authors for their wisdom and dedication to the project. I am also indebted to my Co-Editor, Dr. Amy Y-Y Chen and all of my work colleagues, particularly the dermatology residents (especially Drs. Clay Conner and Elizabeth Usedom) whose support and assistance were essential to bringing this project to fruition. I am eternally grateful for the unending encouragement and inspiration provided by my family (Justin, Sarah and James Trevino and my beloved late parents, Joseph and Felicia Trevino), my church family at Westminster Presbyterian Church in Piqua, Ohio and many dear friends.

Contents

Morphology and Diagnostic Techniques

**Hannah R. Badon, Andrew S. Desrosiers, Robert T. Brodell
and Stephen E. Helms**

Introduction to Morphology

In the United States, it is estimated that 1 of every 3 people is affected by a skin condition at any point in time [1]. The skin is the body's barrier to the outside world and, therefore, may be impacted by UV radiation, irritants, allergens, viruses, bacteria, and arthropods. A damaged barrier can result in rash formation, pruritus, burning sensation, impetigo, cellulitis, and even septicemia or death. Cutaneous signs and symptoms can provide clues as to the possibility of a specific diagnosis related to a wide variety of outdoor hazards so that they can be properly treated or avoided. It is certainly important to separate these conditions from those related to systemic disease.

The diagnosis of skin disease is rooted in the ability to accurately describe dermatological findings. Describing the skin is not just an exercise to promote communication between health care providers. A working knowledge of morphological terminology provides the foundation for developing a differential diagnosis. As the skin is described, the human brain makes connections to the conditions

H. R. Badon (✉) · A. S. Desrosiers
University of Mississippi School of Medicine, Jackson, MS, USA
e-mail: hbadon@umc.edu

A. S. Desrosiers
e-mail: adesrosiers@umc.edu

R. T. Brodell
Department of Dermatology, University of Mississippi Medical Center, Jackson, MS, USA
e-mail: rbrodell@umc.edu

R. T. Brodell
Professor of Pathology, University of Mississippi Medical Center, Jackson, MS, USA

S. E. Helms
Professor of Dermatology, University of Mississippi Medical Center, Jackson, MS, USA
e-mail: sehglh@gmail.com

© Springer Nature Switzerland AG 2020
J. Trevino and A. Y-Y. Chen (eds.), *Dermatological Manual of Outdoor Hazards*,
https://doi.org/10.1007/978-3-030-37782-3_1

associated with or excluded by particular findings. This is a skill that requires study and practice. This chapter defines primary and secondary lesions of the skin as they relate to categorization of specific environmental hazards and also emphasizes the importance of the location and distribution of findings. It also reviews confirmatory tests and warns about common diagnostic pitfalls that affect diagnosis and subsequent choice of treatment. Remember as Yogi Berra said: "If you don't know where you are going, you could wind up someplace else!" [2].

In 2000, the National Institutes of Health (NIH) proposed the development of a dermatology lexicon in order to bring consistency to the study and naming of dermatological diseases [3]. The Dermatology Lexicon Project (DLP) created a vocabulary which includes dermatologic diagnoses, morphologic terminology, laboratory tests, therapies, and procedures [4]. In order to avoid semantic lexical problems, the terms outlined in this chapter will be described using official DLP definitions.

Steps to Dermatologic Diagnosis

The evaluation of a patient with skin findings requires a careful history and physical examination including thorough inspection of the skin. While taking the history, it is imperative to document the onset of the cutaneous lesions, aggravating and alleviating factors, as well as utilization of prescription or over-the-counter remedies and any response to these drugs. A family history pertaining to dermatological or systemic diseases may also be important. Many hazards associated with the natural environment can vary by geographical location and season. Arthropod bites and exposures to plants are naturally more common in warmer months when children and adults are more likely to be outdoors. In the case of arthropod hypersensitivity, it is also important to consider the age of a patient. For instance, newborn patients are much less likely to develop classic fixed urticaria following an arthropod bite due to their naïve immune systems [5]. The clinical finding must also be correlated with travel history and local flora and fauna. In patients already sensitized, poison ivy occurs within 24–48 hours of contact with the plant, and the eruption often lasts for many days [6]. In patients never before allergic to poison ivy, the rash may not appear for several days or up to a week after exposure.

Cutaneous findings are categorized as primary or secondary. The location and distribution of the skin findings should also be documented. The timing of the onset and progression of skin lesions can also provide important information in creating an accurate differential diagnosis. Skin sampling for scabies preparation, KOH preparation, polymerase chain reaction (PCR) and/or cultures for bacteria and viruses may be used to confirm a diagnosis. Other laboratory tests or skin biopsy are less commonly required for the confirmation of a diagnosis. After treatment has been initiated, a follow-up visit may be scheduled to ensure that any evolving clues to diagnosis are identified and any therapy prescribed is working effectively.

Primary Versus Secondary Lesions

Primary lesions are the most important findings in categorizing skin disease. They appear first and often require careful examination to distinguish them from secondary lesions resulting from rubbing, scratching, or senescence. Sometimes they are found in areas where the skin has been undisturbed because it is beyond the patient's reach. Their size, number, color, and associated skin texture should be carefully noted and recorded. Terms used to describe primary lesions are found in Table 1. Primary lesions are defined by specific characteristics. Are the lesions flat or raised, large or small, and solid or fluid-filled? It is often helpful to consider these terms in pairs. For example, patches can be thought of as large macules, and nodules can be thought of as large or deep papules. Hypersensitivity reactions to arthropods are common and generally result in typical reaction patterns that present as fixed, pruritic, urticarial papules (wheals) or, in more severe cases, bullae or patches/plaques with necrosis (Fig. 1a, b) [6]. This can be seen in association with bites from fleas, bedbugs, mosquitoes, lice and field mites. Of course, if the lesions are excoriated or secondarily infected, confirming a diagnosis is more difficult.

Table 1 Primary lesions [4]

Term	DLP proposed definition
Macule	A flat area of skin or mucous membranes with a color different from the surrounding tissue and a diameter generally <0.5 cm; macules may have nonpalpable, fine scales
Patch	A flat area of skin or mucous membranes with a color different from the surrounding tissue and a diameter generally >0.5 cm; patches may have nonpalpable, fine scales
Papule	A discrete, solid, elevated body usually <0.5 cm in diameter, papules are further classified by shape, size, color, and surface change
Plaque	A discrete, solid, elevated body usually broader than it is thick and measuring >0.5 cm in diameter; plaques may be further classified by shape, size, color, and surface change
Vesicle	Fluid-filled cavity or elevation <0.5 cm in diameter; fluid may be clear, serous, or hemorrhagic
Bulla	A fluid-filled blister >0.5 cm in diameter; fluid can be clear, serous, or hemorrhagic
Pustule	A circumscribed elevation that contains pus; pustules are usually <0.5 cm in diameter (see Fig. 2)
Abscess	A localized accumulation of pus in the dermis or subcutaneous tissue; frequently red, warm, and tender
Comedo	An enlarged hair follicular infundibulum primarily containing keratin and lipids with a plugged, dilated, follicular opening (blackhead) or a clinically inapparent follicular opening (whitehead)
Nodule	A dermal or subcutaneous firm, well-defined lesion usually >0.5 cm in diameter
Wheal	An edematous, transitory papule or plaque

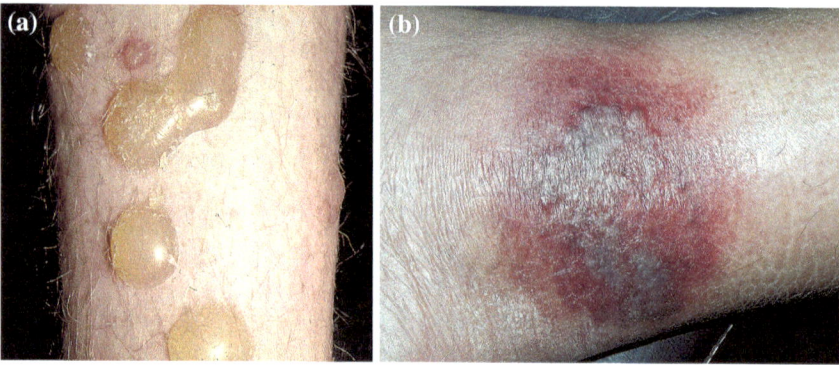

Fig. 1 a Chigger Bites: This patient experienced field mite (chigger) bites and within 2 days developed dozens of 1–3 cm, focally confluent bullae on the lower legs at the sites of each bite. **b** Brown Recluse Spider Bite: A 40-year-old man was working moving boxes in the attic one day before developing this 10 cm diameter patch of tender skin surrounded by a brightly erythematous rim. The black central area has become darker in the past 24 hours

Fig. 2 Pustular psoriasis: A 52-year-old female presented with a 2 week history of erythema and scaling over 90% of her cutaneous surface beginning 1 week after starting vancomycin used to treat "infected insect bites." Close examination reveals hundreds of 0.5–1 mm pustules. Histopathology showed subcorneal pustules with a negative PAS stain

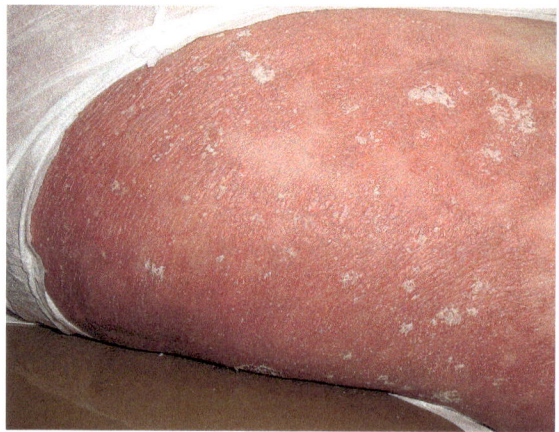

Secondary lesions include scales, excoriations, erosions, ulcers, scars, cutaneous horns, and fissures (Table 2). Secondary lesions are less powerful in making a dermatologic diagnosis. For instance, excoriations can be found in a very broad range of processes. However, these changes can provide clues to the timeline of the process and may support or refute information obtained in the history. If the patient reports no pruritus and denies scratching lesions, the presence of excoriations would prompt more careful probing of the history (Table 2).

Table 2 Secondary lesions [4]

Term	DLP proposed definition
Scales	Small flakes of superficial skin
Excoriations	Abrasions resulting from the scratching or digging of flat or elevated lesions
Erosions	Localized superficial loss of epithelium
Ulcers	Denuded areas of epidermis and some portion or all of the dermis; may be open or covered with a black eschar
Scars	Raised or depressed fibrous lesions caused by trauma or disease
Cutaneous horns	Keratotic projections extending from a skin lesion
Fissures	Cracks that extend through the epidermis into the dermis

Location and Distribution

The location, distribution, and configuration of skin findings can provide clues to a specific diagnosis or differential diagnosis [7]. Location is defined as the specific part or parts of the body that are involved. For example, lesions that appear on the palms and soles of the patient are typical of dyshidrotic eczema or pompholyx, secondary syphilis, or hand, foot, and mouth disease due to coxsackievirus. This type of rash can also be caused by exposure to outdoor hazards such as Rocky Mountain Spotted Fever following a tick bite or allergic contact dermatitis to poison ivy. Distribution refers to the overall pattern of the lesions seen on the surface of the skin; distribution may be symmetrical or asymmetrical. A rash on sun-exposed areas could suggest sunburn (Fig. 3), photo-drug eruption, or polymorphous light eruption. Phytophotodermatitis results from contact with a light sensitizing botanical agent then exposure to ultraviolet light such as the sun. Involvement of skin not protected by clothing is therefore the classic distribution expected with

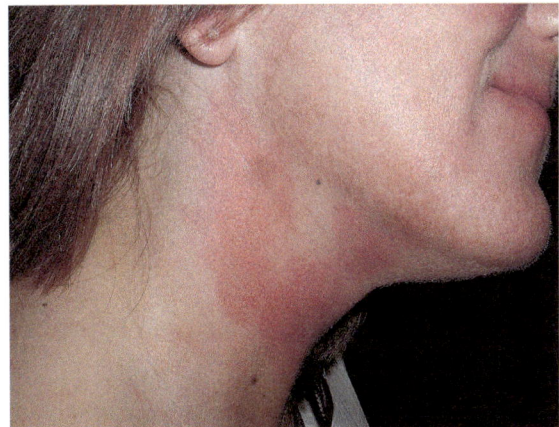

Fig. 3 Sunburn: A 32-year-old female fell asleep in the sun after quickly applying sunscreen to her face (sun protection factor (SPF) 30). The face and a small patch on the right neck visible in this image were spared because of the protective effects of sunscreen

dermatoses due to hazardous arthropods and plants. Configuration refers to the grouping of lesions. Terms pertaining to lesion configuration include annular, linear, targetoid, and many others. Recognizing the configuration of the lesions can be extremely helpful in pinpointing the correct diagnosis (Table 3) [8]. The presence of a pruritic, papulovesicular rash with linearity is one of the most powerful findings to suggest the diagnosis of allergic contact dermatitis (Fig. 4). This dermatitis can be caused by skin exposure to the chemical urushiol contained in the leaves of plants in the Anacardiaceae family in the genus *Toxicodendron* such as poison ivy, oak, and sumac [6]. A grouping of fixed urticarial papules associated

Table 3 Lesion configuration [8]

Configuration	Definition	Disease example
Annular	Lesions in a ring	Tinea corporis
Digitate	Lesions in the shape of a fingertip	Mycosis fungoides
Grouped or herpetiform	Many lesions appearing in a well-defined, small area	Herpes simplex infections
Linear	Lesions grouped in a linear formation	Contact dermatitis
Serpiginous	Lesions appearing in snake-like formations	Cutaneous larva migrans
Targetoid	Lesions appearing in the shape of a target	Erythema multiforme
Zosteriform	Lesions grouped in one dermatome	Herpes zoster (shingles)

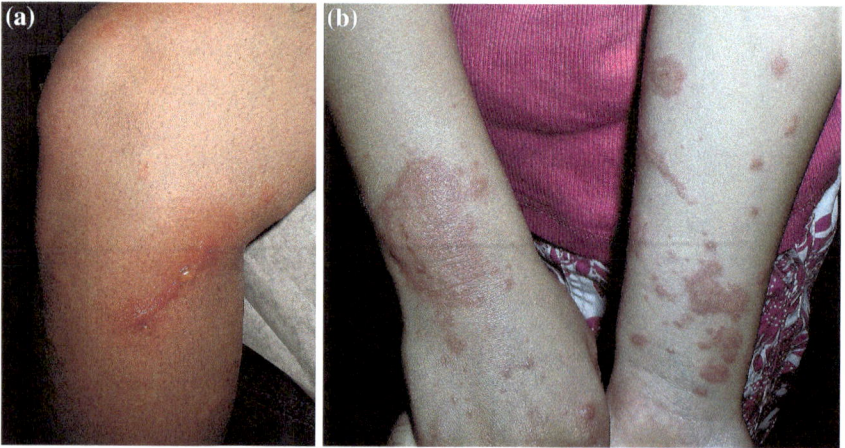

Fig. 4 a Poison Ivy Dermatitis: This 22-year-old woman presented with a linear, papulovesicular eruption on the right medial lower leg just below the knee with several 2–3 mm papulovesicular papules elsewhere on the lower legs 4 days after "hiking in the woods." **b** Poison Ivy Dermatitis: This 40-year-old female presented with erythematous papules and plaques with focal linearity. Tiny papulovesicles are noted in some areas

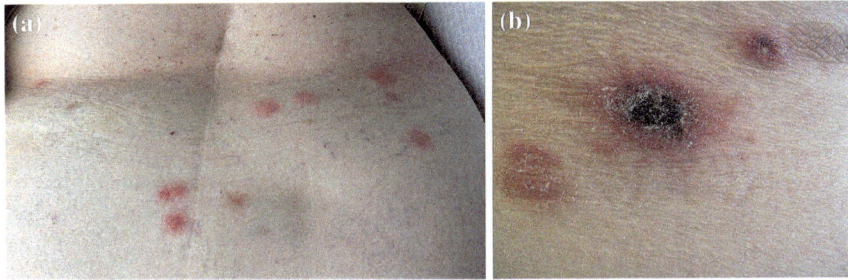

Fig. 5 a Bed Bug bites. This 50-year-old patient developed these 6–8 mm diameter "fixed" urticarial lesions after sleeping in a hotel the night before. She brought in a "bug" she found on the sheets when she woke up which proved to be cimex lectularius (bed bug). **b** Bed Bug Bites with secondary changes: A 26-year-old patient developed these bed-bug bites after staying in a hotel. Note the "breakfast, lunch and dinner" grouping. Scratching the central lesion led to crusting with a rim of erythema. The other two lesions show a "fixed urticaria" edematous appearance. (Used with permission of Whitney High, MD, University of Colorado, Departments of Dermatology and Pathology)

with insect bites is often referred to as "breakfast, lunch, and dinner" sign (Fig. 5a and b).

Confirmatory Testing

A potassium hydroxide (KOH) preparation is a simple, reproducible, and cost-effective method to confirm the diagnosis of a suspected fungal infection. Scale is obtained by lightly "scraping" scaly skin or a portion of crumbly, thickened nail plate onto a glass slide. After a cover slip or cover glass is placed on the slide, KOH 10% solution is added, and the slide is gently heated over an alcohol lamp to clear the keratin and allow hyphae to be easily visualized. The condenser of the microscope should be lowered prior to searching for hyphae. Utilizing stains such as Chicago blue or chlorazol black E colors the hyphae, making them easier to visualize (Fig. 6a, b, c). Dimethyl sulfoxide is occasionally added to the KOH solution to permit rapid clearing of keratin without heating [9].

Another useful, simple, bedside test is the scabies preparation. This is best used in conjunction with the burrow ink test. Water soluble fountain pen ink is rubbed on suspected sites such as the finger webs, wrists, elbows, or axillae. An alcohol swab is used to wipe away any excess ink. In patients with scabies, an ink-filled burrow created by the mite tunneling through the stratum corneum may be visible (Fig. 7a and b) [10]. After applying mineral oil to the skin, a 15 blade is used to unroof the burrow by lightly scraping the skin until the inked burrow is no longer visible and the contents of the burrow are floating in the oil. This oil is then applied to a glass slide, a cover slip is placed, and the slide is then examined for

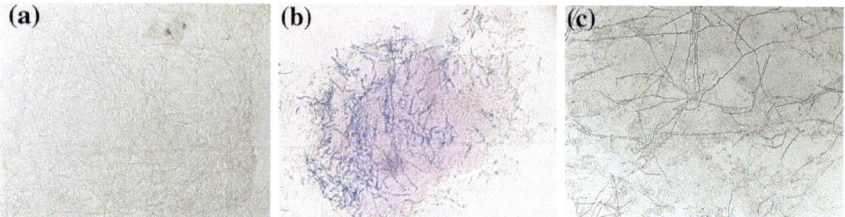

Fig. 6 **a** Tinea: Hyphae are seen crisscrossing this field. Their length distinguishes them from the cell membranes of keratinocytes (KOH, 100x). **b** Tinea: Chicago blue mixed with KOH stains fungal cell walls highlighting the hyphae with a blue color that stand out from unstained keratinocyte (Chicago blue KOH, 100x). **c** Tinea: Chlorazole black E mixed with KOH stains hyphae black causing them to stand out from the membranes of background keratinocytes cleared by the KOH (Chlorazole black E, 100x)

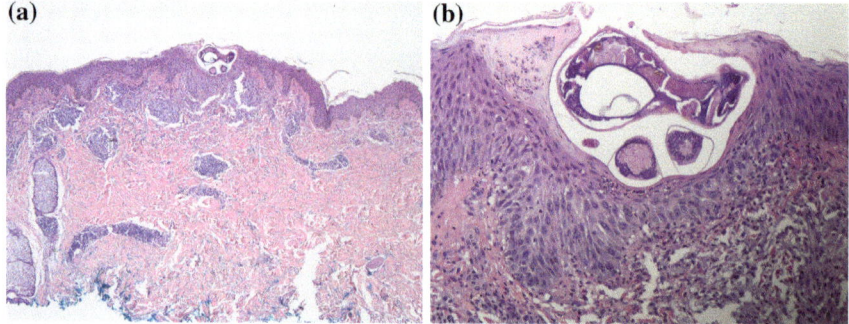

Fig. 7 **a** Scabies: This photomicrograph demonstrates a subcorneal burrow containing a scabies mite. Underlying mixed inflammation including lymphocytes and numerous eosinophils is seen. Unfortunately, many biopsy specimens from patients with scabies do not show burrows or mites making the scabies preparation the preferred diagnostic method (H&E, 40x). **b** Scabies: This closer view shows the chitinous exoskeleton with spicules, GI tract, and mouth parts of the scabies mite (H&E, 400x)

scabies mites, eggs, and scybala (feces) (Fig. 8). A substantial case series reported that the ideal location for the burrow ink test is the medial aspect of the hypothenar area [11].

Wood's lamp testing is commonly used to evaluate disorders of pigmentation, both hypopigmentation and hyperpigmentation. This light source emits wavelengths between 320 and 400 nm with a peak at 365 nm [12]. Filtered light from the Wood's lamp is absorbed by the skin, and radiation of a longer wavelength is emitted by fluorescence, which is best observed in a completely dark room. Non-diseased skin appears blue, depigmented skin (vitiligo) appears white, and hypopigmentation (e.g. post-inflammatory hypopigmentation) blends into the blue coloration of surrounding skin (Fig. 9a and b). Additionally, Wood's lamp can be used for the diagnosis of certain bacterial or fungal infections.

Fig. 8 Scabies: An 8-legged scabies mite is identified in a scabies prep

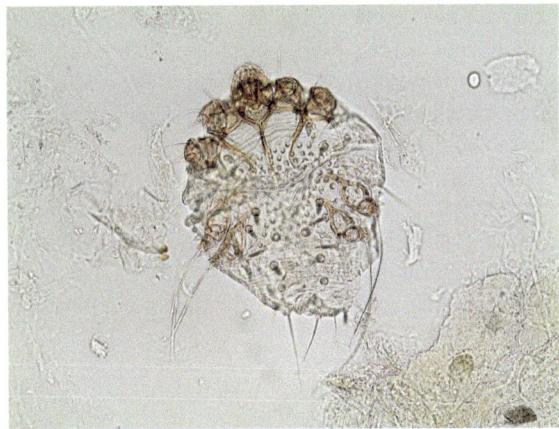

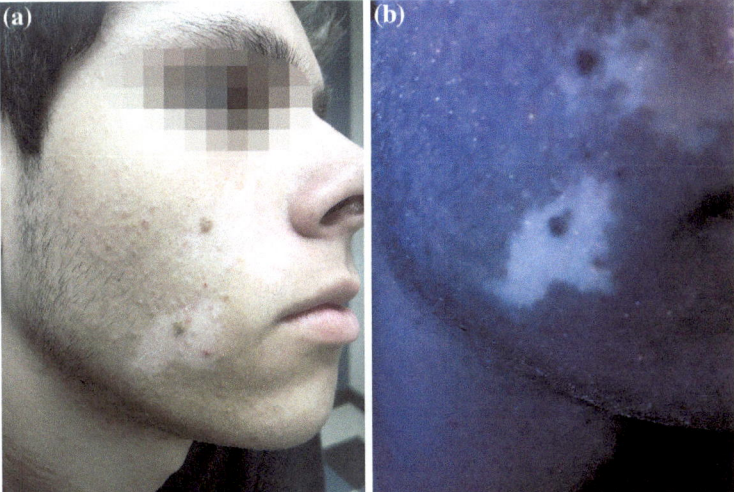

Fig. 9 **a** Halo nevi: This 21-year-old patient presented with a 4-month history of halos appearing around two nevi each 4 mm in diameter on the right cheek. **b** Halo Nevi: The halo is accentuated under a Wood's Lamp providing evidence of complete depigmentation in the skin surrounding the mole

Pseudomonas infections under the nail plate or in impetiginized skin appear green. *Corynebacterium minutissimum* infections, such as pitted keratolysis or erythrasma, exhibit coral red fluorescence [12].

In the context of a patient who owns pets (e.g. cats, dogs, rabbits) and develops pruritic red bumps on the arms, chest, or abdomen, *Cheyletiella* mites may be suspected. The best confirmatory test when suspecting *Cheyletiella* is conducted on the pet, not the patient. A cellophane tape preparation reveals the larval or adult form of the species. Similarly, lice infestations are generally identified by examining the seams of clothing not the patient's skin. Head and pubic lice can be identified by the naked eye or utilizing a hand lens. When questioning whether or not hair casts or nits are present, microscopic examination of involved hairs (trichoscopy) will reveal the nits cemented to hair shafts in patients with head lice.

A skin biopsy is generally not the initial approach to confirming a diagnosis in conditions caused by outdoor hazards. A KOH preparation, scabies prep, or Wood's lamp exam are much less expensive and less invasive than a biopsy. Of course, individuals who develop skin cancer from outdoor UV exposure should have a biopsy to confirm the diagnosis and plan appropriate treatment.

Diagnostic Pitfalls

Unfortunately, health care providers are sometimes overconfident and jump to conclusions when making a diagnosis. After a thorough history and careful clinical examination of the skin, health care providers should carefully consider a broad differential diagnosis and then perform appropriate tests to narrow down these options to a final working diagnosis. Defining a diagnosis through use of

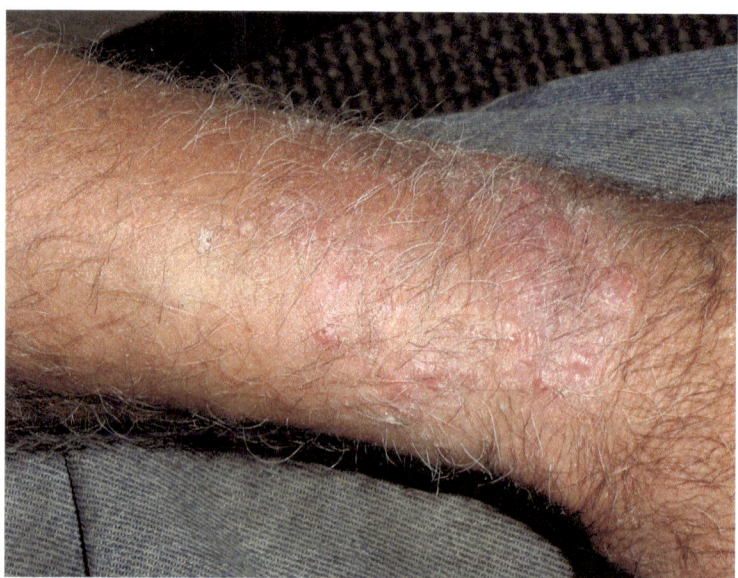

Fig. 10 Tinea incognito: This 40-year-old man had a 2 cm diameter scaling rash on the left forearm. Treatment with Clobetasol 0.05% cream twice daily for 3 months. The patch expanded to 10 cm in diameter. Mild scaling and erythema with a dozen 1.5 mm acneiform papules is noted. The typical accentuated peripheral scale of tinea corporis is not present because of the anti-inflammatory effects of the topical steroid

therapeutic trials or a "shot-gun" approach using multiple treatments to cover all possibilities often leads to an increased risk of side effects and failed therapy. For example, when tinea corporis is mistaken for "dermatitis" and treated utilizing topical steroids without performing a KOH preparation, tinea incognito can be produced (Fig. 10). The steroid lowers local immunity leading to proliferation of the superficial fungal infection in a manner that obscures classic clinical features. This makes it more difficult to make the correct diagnosis at future visits [13].

Conclusion

As the interface between humans and the outside world (e.g. plants and arthropods), the skin provides visual clues to determine the likely diagnosis and proper treatment. With practice, a differential diagnosis can be built and narrowed by considering morphology, location, distribution, and categorical groupings. The correct diagnosis is made when this differential diagnosis is further evaluated with confirmatory testing when appropriate.

Disclosures   None of the authors have relevant conflicts of interest.

References

1. Johnson ML. Defining the burden of skin disease in the United States—a historical perspective. J Invest Dermatol. 2004;9:108–10.
2. Gorman M. Yogi Berra's most memorable sayings; 2015. https://www.newsweek.com/most-memorable-yogi-isms-375661. Accessed 13 Feb 2019.
3. Goldsmith L, Papier A. Fighting babel with precise definitions of knowledge. J Invest Dermatol. 2010;11:2527–30.
4. Dermatology Lexicon Project. Morphologic terminology; 2002. https://people.rit.edu/grh-fad/DLP2/index.html. Accessed 18 Nov 2018.
5. Hernandez R, Cohen B. Insect bite-induced hypersensitivity and the SCRATCH principles: a new approach to papular urticaria. Pediatrics. 2006;118:189–96.
6. Yesul K, Longenecker A, Mahmoud E, et al. Urushiol patch test using the TRUE TEST system. Dermatitis. 2018;29:127–131.
7. Armstrong A. Approach to the clinical dermatologic diagnosis. In: Corona R editor. UpToDate. Retrieved 20 Dec 2018, from https://www.uptodate.com/contents/approach-to-the-clinical-dermatologic-diagnosis#H7.
8. Brodell RT, Dolohanty LB, Helms SE. Approach to the diagnosis of skin disease. In: Singh A, editor. Scientific American Medicine. Toronto: Decker;2017. https://doi.org/10.2310/7900.1228, https://www.deckerip.com/decker/medicine/chapter/46/#approach-to-the-diagnosis-of-skin-disease.
9. Martin A, Kobayashi G. Yeast infestations: candidiasis, pityriasis (tinea) versicolor. In Fitzpatrick T, Eisen, A, Wolff K, et al editors. Dermatology in general medicine, 4th ed. New York: McGraw-Hill;1993. pp. 2462–67.
10. Leung V, Miller M. Detection of scabies: a systematic review of diagnostic methods. Can J Infect Dis Med Microbiol. 2011;22:143–6.

11. Woodley D, Saurat JH. The burrow ink test and the scabies mite. J Am Acad Dermatol. 1981;4:715–22.
12. Sharma S, Sharma A. Robert Williams Wood: pioneer of invisible light. Photodermatol Photo. 2016;32:60–5.
13. Polilli E, Fazii P, Ursini T, et al. Tinea incognito caused by microsporum gypseum in a patient with advanced HIV infection: a case report. Case Rep Dermatol. 2011;3:55–9.

Plant-Induced Urticaria

Preeti Jhorar and Wyatt J. Andrasik

Introduction

Urticaria is an extremely common skin eruption that occurs in up to 20% of the population [1]. The term 'urticaria' is originally derived from the plant genus, *Urtica*, which encompasses the ubiquitous stinging nettle, known for causing classic urticarial wheal-and-flare reaction [2]. Certain plants can cause contact urticaria, referring to the abrupt onset of the pruritic skin eruption following external contact with a substance [3, 4]. Plant-induced urticaria is relatively uncommon and is divided into two pathogenetically distinct types—immunologic contact urticaria (ICU) caused by IgE-mediated release of vasoactive mediators from mast cells, and non-immunologic contact urticaria (NICU), also referred to as toxin-mediated urticaria, caused by direct inoculation of irritant chemicals from sharp hairs on leaves and stems [5]. Like all forms of urticaria, both types present with an eruption composed of wheals, well-defined superficial swellings of dermis characterized by pink to erythematous papules or plaques with surrounding red flare.

Immunologic Contact Urticaria

ICU, while less common than NICU, has potential for serious sequela such as chronic dermatitis, oropharyngeal swelling, systemic symptoms, and anaphylaxis [3, 5]. Most reactions consist of localized wheals that appear within 30 min of contact and clear completely within hours; however, generalized urticaria has been

P. Jhorar · W. J. Andrasik (✉)
Wright State University Boonshoft School of Medicine, Dayton, OH, USA
e-mail: wyatt.andrasik@gmail.com

P. Jhorar
e-mail: preetijhorar@yahoo.com

© Springer Nature Switzerland AG 2020
J. Trevino and A. Y-Y. Chen (eds.), *Dermatological Manual of Outdoor Hazards*,
https://doi.org/10.1007/978-3-030-37782-3_2

reported [3]. In rare cases, ICU may progress to involve the respiratory, gastrointestinal, and cardiovascular systems requiring emergent medical care (see Table 1) [3]. Repeated urticarial eruptions may eventually evolve into a chronic or recurrent eczematous dermatitis termed, protein contact dermatitis (PCD), which typically affects the hands and forearms [3]. Individuals affected by ICU are also predisposed to oral allergy syndrome (OAS), a mucosal contact urticaria seen in people cross-sensitized to pollen and similar allergens in fruits, vegetables, and nuts [3, 6]. Eating foods that contain these homologous allergens cause immediate oral cavity itching, stinging, and pain that lasts for minutes after swallowing [6, 7]. Some attacks may progress to swelling of the lips, tongue, and soft palate, but rarely progress to anaphylaxis [6].

Theoretically, any plant can induce ICU, but common culprits include plants from families Asteracea, Apiaceae, Agavaceae, and Moraceae [3]. Examples of reported urticants include fruits (i.e. apple, banana, lemon, tomato), vegetables (i.e. carrot, celery, lettuce, onion, potato), herbs and spices (i.e. dill, parsley), decorative plants (i.e. bishop's weed, chrysanthemum, peace lily, tulip, weeping fig, yucca), trees and shrubs (i.e. birch, common dogwood), grains (i.e. barley, wheat), and nuts (i.e. pecan, walnut) [3, 5, 8–11]. A list of plants that have been reported to cause ICU can be found in Table 2.

Table 1 Stages of contact urticaria syndrome

Contact urticaria syndrome	
Stage 1	Localized urticaria; non-specific symptoms (i.e. pruritus, burning, tingling)
Stage 2	Generalized urticaria with or without angioedema
Stage 3	Systemic involvement (i.e. rhinoconjunctivitis, bronchospasm, orolaryngeal, gastrointestinal symptoms)
Stage 4	Anaphylactic shock

Table 2 Plants that cause ICU [3, 5, 8–11, 14, 16, 24, 25]

Plants causing immunologic contact urticaria		
Category	Common name	
Fruits	Apple	Olive
	Apricot	Orange
	Banana	Peach
	Fig	Pear
	Grapefruit	Pineapple
	Kiwi	Plum
	Lemon	Strawberry
	Melon	Tomato

(continued)

Table 2   (continued)

Plants causing immunologic contact urticaria		
Category	Common name	
Vegetables	Artichoke	Green pepper
	Asparagus	Horseradish
	Cabbage	Lettuce
	Carrot	Mushroom
	Cauliflower	Onion
	Celery	Parsnips
	Chives	Potato
	Cucumber	Spinach
	Eggplant	Watercress
	Endive	
Herbs and spices	Chicory	Dill
	Cinnamon	Garlic
	Coriander	Mustard
	Cress	Paprika
	Cumin	Parsley
Decorative plants	American aloe	Transvaal daisy
	Bishop's weed	Tulip
	Chrysanthemum	Weeping fig
	Daffodil	Yucca
	Peace lily	
Trees and shrubs	Balsam of Peru	Limba
	Birch	Sap
	Brazil nut tree	Sapele
	Coffee	Singleseed hawthorn
	Common dogwood	Obeche
	European larch	Teak
	Henna	Western red cedar
	Indian rosewood	
Grains	Barley	Rye
	Cornstarch	Wheat
	Oat	
Nuts	Almond	Pecan
	Hazelnut	Walnut
	Peanut	
Other	Alfalfa	Red clover
	Golden crownbeard	Swiss cheese plant
	Hops	

Non-immunologic Contact Urticaria

Non-immunologic contact urticaria (NICU) occurs more frequently and presents similarly to ICU with onset of wheals occurring within minutes of contact. Eruptions are generally mild and self-limiting, although subjective symptoms such as paresthesia may last hours, even after skin findings resolve [12]. In cases involving the Gympie-Gympie (*Dendrocnide moroides*), urticaria, paresthesia, and pain can last months and require hospitalization [13]. Plants from many families cause NICU, but none are more notorious than the nettle family (Urticaceae) which includes the stinging nettles. Other common families include the spurge family (Euphorbiaceae), water-leaf family (Hydrophyllaceae), and Loasaceae family [14, 15]. A list of plants that cause NICU can be found in Table 3.

Other Causes of Contact Urticaria

Urticarial reactions caused by algae, cyanobacteria, fungi, and lichen (composite organisms composed of fungi and algae) are often wrongfully attributed to plants. Eruptions caused by these offenders belong to different taxonomic kingdoms and are not discussed in this chapter.

Epidemiology

Urticaria is among the most common types of skin manifestations. Plant-induced urticaria is far less common, but the exact prevalence is difficult to estimate as many cases undoubtedly go unreported.

ICU is relatively uncommon, especially in those without extensive, occupational exposures to plants and plant products. Studies estimate that almost 95% of non-latex ICU is work-related [4]. The strongest predisposing factors are frequent contact with plants seen in gardeners, greenhouse workers, and florists, as well as frequent contact with fruits, vegetables and spices seen in food processors, food handlers, caterers, and cooks [3, 16–18]. Other risk factors include atopy, sensitive skin prone to eczema, and underlying dermatitis, especially hand dermatitis [3, 16, 18]. Up to 22% with ICU go on to develop PCD and suffer significant work-related consequences such as changing work tasks and requesting longer sick leave [18]. Eventually, over 60% of those with PCD need to change jobs [18].

NICU is the most common type of lant-induced contact urticaria because it occurs without the need for previous sensitization and anyone exposed can be affected [5]. Species of the nettle family are a major cause of NICU and can be found worldwide [12, 19]. The stinging nettle, *Urtica dioica*, is the most common cause of NICU in the United States and United Kingdom [12, 19–21].

Table 3 Plants that cause NICU [5, 13–15, 33–35]

Plants causing non-immunologic contact urticaria			
Family	Scientific name	Common name	Distribution
Urticaceae	*Urtica dioica*	Stinging nettle	Worldwide
	Urtica urens	Dwarf nettle	Worldwide
	Urtica pilulifera	Roman nettle	Worldwide
	Laportea canadensis	Canadian wood nettle	North America
	Dendrocnide moroides	Gympie-Gympie	Australian rainforest; Southeast Asia
	Dendrocnide excelsa	Giant stinging tree	Australian rainforest; Southeast Asia
	Dendrocnide photinophylla	Shining-leaved stinging tree	Australian rainforest
Euphorbiaceae	*Euphorbia characias*	Mediterranean spurge	Mediterranean basin
	Cnidoscolus stimulosus	Spurge nettle	Central America; South America
	Cnidoscolus megacanthus	–	Central America; South America
	Cnidoscolus urens	Bull nettle	Central America; South America
	Cnidoscolus texanus	Texas bullnettle	Central America; South America
	Tragia lessertiana	–	Worldwide
	Dalechampia stipulacea	–	Worldwide
	Ricinus communis	Castor oil plant	North America, Europe, Asia, Africa
Hydrophyllaceae	*Wigandia urens*	–	United States; southern Australia; Europe; South Africa
Loasaceae	*Blumenbachia spp.*	–	United States; Mexico; South America
	Caiophora spp.	–	United States; Mexico; South America
	Loasa spp.	–	United States; Mexico; South America

Classification

ICU is caused by IgE-mediated release of vasoactive mediators from mast cells. NICU is caused by direct inoculation of irritant chemicals from sharp hairs, termed trichomes, on leaves and stems of plants (see Figs. 1 and 2) [5].

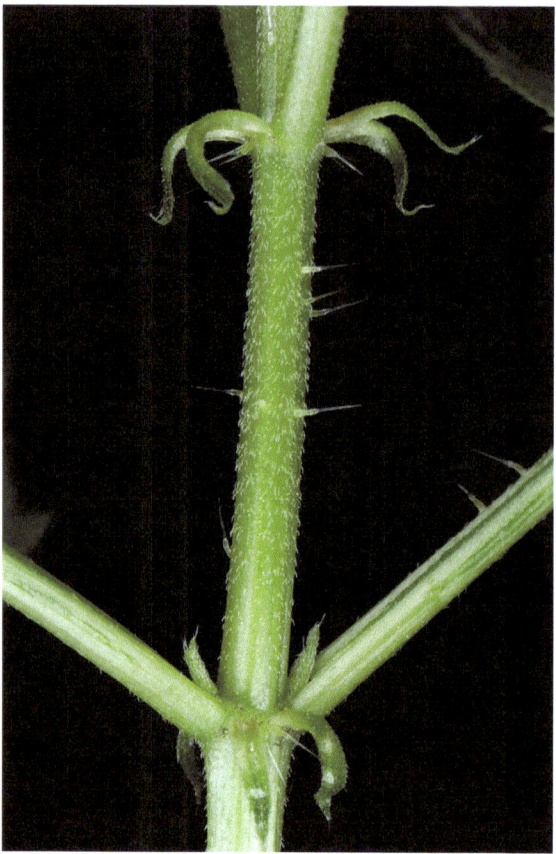

Fig. 1 Close-up of trichomes on stem of a stinging nettle (*Urtica dioica*). Doug Goldman, Hosted by the USDA-NRCS PLANTS Database [21]

Clinical Features

Clinical features of plant-induced contact urticaria vary greatly. Most reactions present with a localized eruption of wheals. Lesions range from a few millimeters to more than 10 cm in size and from a few to many in number. Associated symptoms often include pruritus, burning, stinging, and tingling [5]. Some cases may only present with non-specific dermatitis manifesting as erythema or with subjective symptoms of pruritus, tingling, or burning without overt clinical findings [5]. This heterogeneity in clinical presentation makes it a challenge to diagnose plant-induced contact urticaria.

Immunologic Contact Urticaria

ICU requires prior sensitization to the allergen and therefore, is more common in patients with atopy and extensive, repeat exposures to plants [3, 16, 18]. Raw

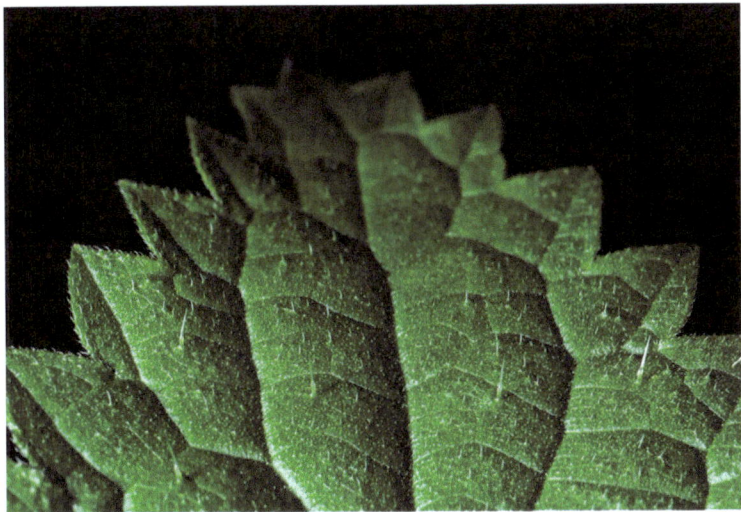

Fig. 2 Close-up of trichomes on leaf of a stinging nettle (*Urtica dioica*). Doug Goldman, Hosted by the USDA-NRCS PLANTS Database [21]

foods are thought to be more allergenic and sometimes, but not always, processing, cooking, and deep-freezing can reduce their allergenicity [22, 23].

Clinical features vary significantly from non-specific signs and symptoms such as pruritus, burning, tingling, and erythema to anaphylaxis. While most reactions consist of localized wheals that appear within 30 min of contact and clear completely within hours, some may progress to generalized urticaria or involve the respiratory, gastrointestinal, and cardiovascular systems [3]. Given the array of clinical findings, the term 'contact urticaria syndrome' has been proposed and is divided into four stages based on severity of symptoms (see Table 1) [3].

Pathogenesis

ICU is IgE-mediated and requires prior sensitization with the allergen. After sensitization, repeat exposure to the allergen causes immediate degranulation and release of mast cell mediators such as histamine. Other inflammatory compounds such as prostaglandins and leukotrienes are thought to play a role as well [5].

Plants Causing ICU

Plants that commonly cause ICU include fruits (i.e. apple, banana, lemon, tomato), vegetables (i.e. carrot, celery, lettuce, onion, potato), herbs and spices (i.e. dill, parsley), decorative plants (i.e. bishop's weed, chrysanthemum, peace lily, tulip, weeping fig, yucca), trees and shrubs (i.e. birch, common dogwood), grains (i.e. barley, wheat), and nuts (i.e. pecan, walnut) [3, 5, 8–11]. A list of plants that have been reported to cause ICU is found in Table 2.

Other Manifestations of ICU

There are several other manifestations of ICU that deserve special mention—protein contact dermatitis and oral allergy syndrome.

Protein contact dermatitis (PCD) is a form of chronic or recurrent eczematous dermatitis that typically affects the hands and forearms [3]. Most cases are seen in food handlers that come in contact with allergens under prolonged, wet conditions, although there are reports involving non-edible plants [18, 26]. Other risk factors include those with a history of atopy [26]. Upon contact, culprit protein allergens pass through the skin barrier and sensitize the immune system, making patients susceptible to the IgE-mediated reaction when subsequently exposed to the same allergen [3, 26]. Patients present with acute on chronic dermatitis manifesting as erythema, urticaria, and vesicular eruptions of the fingers and hands, sometimes extending to the forearms [3, 26]. Subjective symptoms such as pruritus or tingling and chronic paronychia are also possible [3, 26]. Approximately half of patients with occupation-related PCD can have concomitant occupational airway disease; hence, patients suspected to have PCD should always be asked about respiratory symptoms [27]. A wide range of plants are responsible for causing PCD. Common culprits include kiwi, pineapple, tomato, fig, carrot, celery, potato, onion, dill, and garlic [3, 28].

Oral allergy syndrome (OAS) is an IgE-mediated mucosal contact urticaria in people cross-sensitized to pollen and similar allergens in fruits, vegetables, and nuts [3, 6]. It occurs more commonly after ingestion of uncooked fruits and raw vegetables, and in those with a history of atopy [7, 29]. Eating foods that contain these homologous allergens causes immediate oral cavity itching, stinging, pain, and throat tightness that lasts for minutes after swallowing [6, 7]. Some attacks may go on to cause swelling of the lips, tongue and soft palate, and rarely progress to anaphylaxis [6]. While symptoms are usually limited to the oral mucosa, if the allergen is ingested in large quantities, patients can experience gastrointestinal symptoms [29]. Commonly implicated plants are those that share allergens with pollen, ragweed, or grass such as banana, tomato, peach, melon, celery, onion, garlic, almond, hazelnut, and peanut [29, 30]. Thoroughly cooked food items can sometimes be tolerated by patients with OAS, but this is not always the case, especially with cooked celery and roasted hazelnuts [31, 32].

OAS is distinct from simple food allergies where symptoms develop due to direct sensitization to culprit food proteins rather than cross-reactivity between food proteins and inhalant allergies [29].

Non-immunologic Contact Urticaria

Clinical features of NICU primarily consist of localized wheals at the site of contact that occur within minutes of exposure. Subjective symptoms such as burning, pain, and paresthesia commonly accompany skin whealing, but may be present without cutaneous manifestations. Eruptions are generally mild and self-limiting, resolving within several hours. Rarely, subjective symptoms may last days to months, even after skin findings resolve [12]. Systemic symptoms are uncommon, but reactions involving *Dendrocnide spp.* can be severe and life-threatening [13].

Pathogenesis

NICU is caused by direct contact with trichomes on stems and leaves of inciting plants. Trichomes are composed of two parts—a proximal fine tube-like hair and distal bulb [12]. Upon contact, the distal bulb breaks off and the remaining trichome penetrates the skin, releasing a cocktail of irritant chemicals such as histamine, serotonin, acetylcholine, and formic acid [33]. Thus, the mechanism is thought to be a synergistic effect of both mechanical and chemical irritation [19].

Plants Causing NICU

Plants from four families cause NICU and include the nettle family (Urticaceae), spurge family (Euphorbiaceae) , water-leaf family (Hydrophyllaceae), and Loasaceae family (Figs. 3, 4, 5 and 6) [14, 15]. The ubiquitous nettle family is responsible for most cases of NICU. The stinging nettle, *Urtica dioica*, is the most common cause of NICU in the United States and United Kingdom (Figs. 3 and 4) [12, 19–21]. A list of plants known to cause NICU can be found in Table 3.

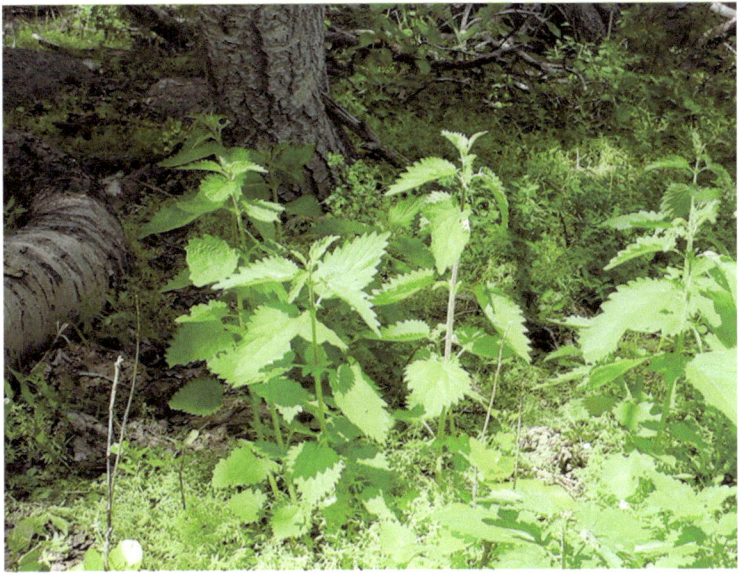

Fig. 3 Stinging nettle (*Urtica dioica*). These plants stand 1–2 feet tall and are commonly found in moist woods and along roadsides. Sheri Hagwood, Hosted by the USDA-NRCS PLANTS Database [21]

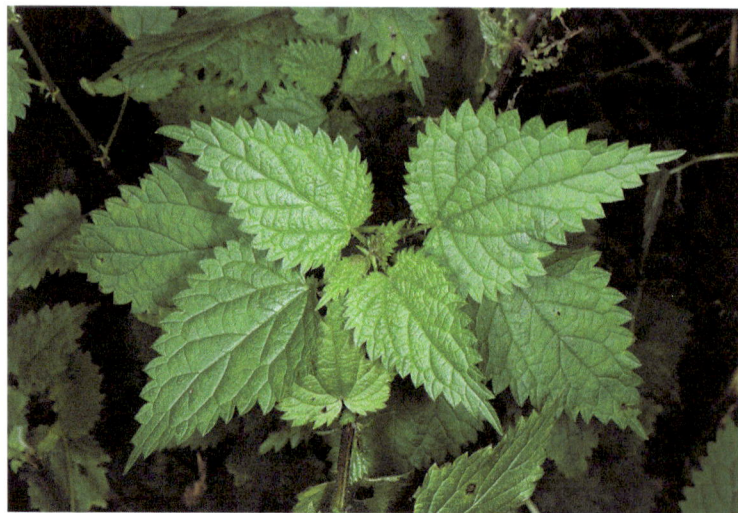

Fig. 4 Characteristic saw-toothed, heart shaped leaves of the stinging nettle (*Urtica dioica*). Doug Goldman, Hosted by the USDA-NRCS PLANTS Database [21]

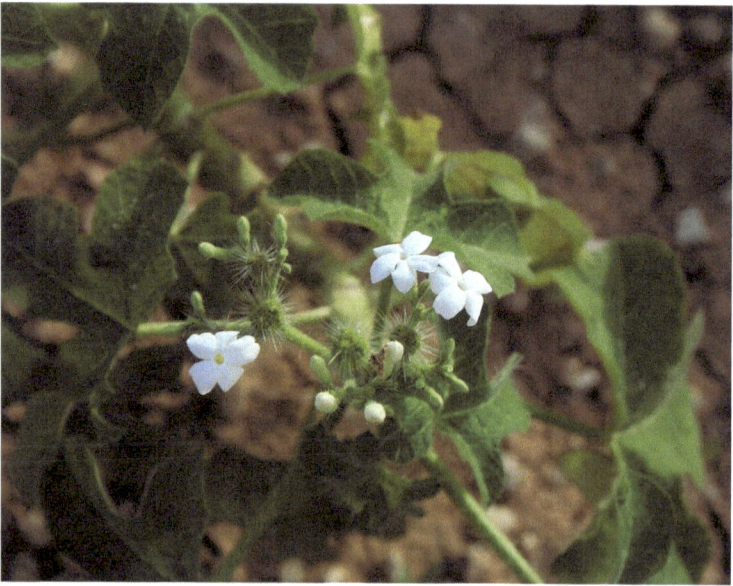

Fig. 5 Euphorbiaceae family, *Cnidoscolus urens*. Photo by Franz Xaver https://commons.wiki-media.org/w/index.php?curid=65659757

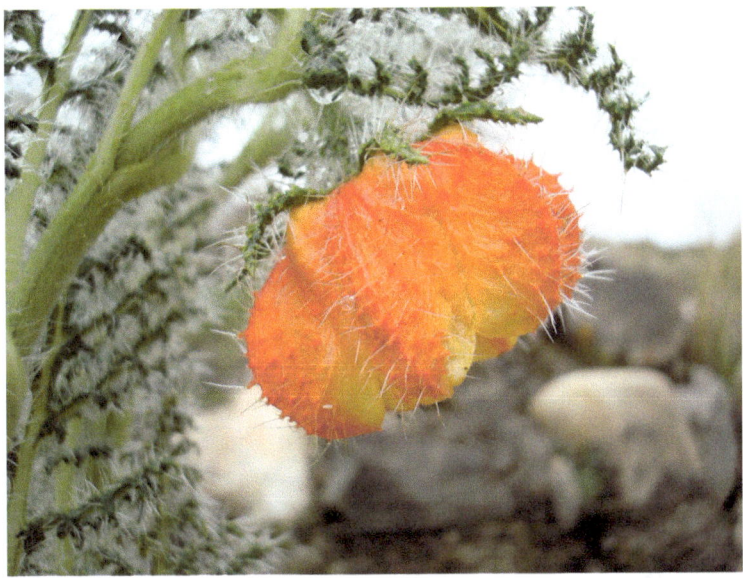

Fig. 6 Close-up of Loasaceae flower. Photo by Olga Lidia Paredes https://commons.wikimedia.org/w/index.php?curid=26538729

Diagnosis

Diagnosis should begin with a detailed history and clinical examination of the skin. If contact urticaria is suspected, additional testing may be performed to confirm the diagnosis. Ideally, nonsteroidal anti-inflammatory drugs and antihistamines should be avoided during testing and in the 3–4 days prior to testing [4].

Immunologic Contact Urticaria

Given that ICU is an IgE-mediated reaction, a skin prick test (SPT) with fresh plant material is the test of choice [3]. Commercial preparations of protein allergens can be used, but few are available for plants and are less reliable than fresh preparations [5, 29]. If there is a history or serious concern for anaphylaxis to the suspected plant, a graded approach to testing should be taken (Fig. 7).

Specific IgE tests such as the radioallergosorbent (RAST) test or Immuno-CAP test for known proteins are useful, when available, but are costly and many plant protein allergens have not been identified [3]. When specific IgE tests are not possible, an open application test should be performed by applying fresh plant material to a 3 cm × 3 cm area of hairless, intact skin for several minutes [4, 5]. Skin

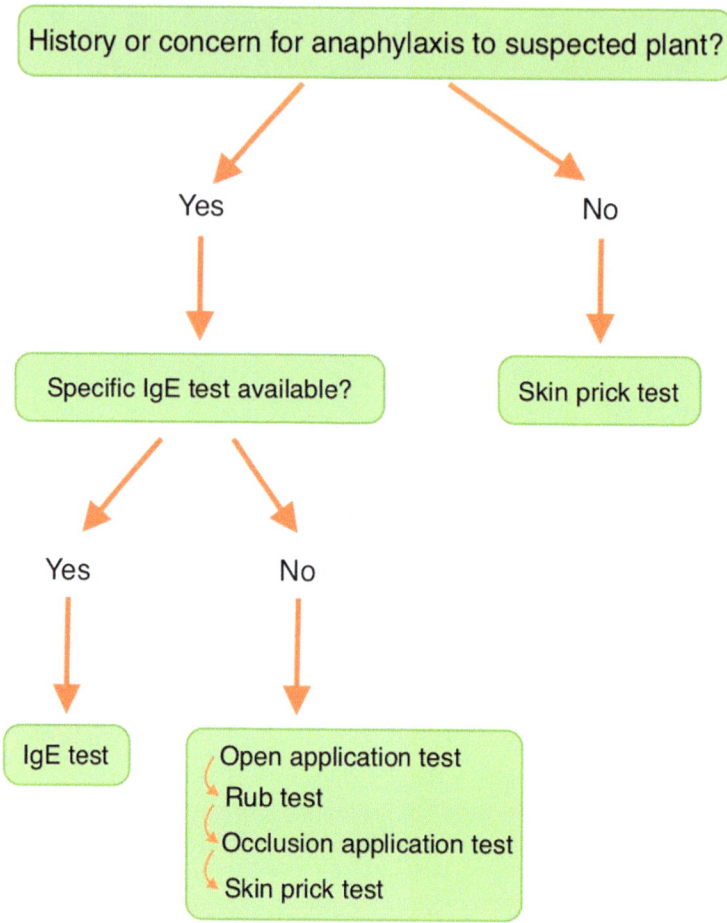

Fig. 7 Graded diagnostic approach to ICU

should be observed for 60 min, looking for signs of erythema, edema, or wheal-ing [5]. Observations should be recorded every 10–15 min to avoid false nega-tive results [5]. If no reaction is appreciated, the test should be repeated on mildly affected or previously affected skin, although results may be more difficult to interpret [3–5]. Oftentimes, open application testing may be negative due to poor penetration of the large plant proteins [5]. To enhance skin penetration, a rub test can be performed by gently rubbing fresh plant material several times over the test area [3]. Again, the skin should be observed for 60 min, checking for a positive reaction periodically. If no reaction is appreciated, the test should be repeated on mildly affected or previously affected skin [3–5]. Before escalating to a SPT, an occlusion application test should be performed by applying fresh plant material to the skin and occluding with porous tape or plastic wrap for 20 min and observing for an additional 60 min [5]. Test materials should be removed immediately after signs of a positive reaction to avoid progression to systemic symptoms [5]. If no reaction is appreciated, the test should be repeated on mildly affected or previously affected skin.

A SPT can be done by applying fresh plant material to the skin and passing a 1 mm needle through the material into the epidermis [5]. Histamine dihydrochloride solution (1–10 mg/ml) should be used as a positive control and a drop of physiologic saline as a negative control [5]. Given the potential for serious systemic reactions, tests should be done in a facility with adequate resuscitation equipment and trained personnel [3, 4].

When diagnosing PCD, the same diagnostic approach should be used [3]. When diagnosing OAS, a detailed history is of utmost importance. Patients should endorse oropharyngeal symptoms with ingestion of certain raw fruits or vegetables as well as a history of pollen-associated allergies [29]. A SPT with fresh plant material is the test of choice, although IgE tests for many indicted proteins are also available. An oral food challenge is reasonable, but generally unnecessary.

Non-immunologic Contact Urticaria

The diagnostic approach to NICU is much simpler as there is minimal risk for serious systemic reactions. In many cases, testing is not required, and a diagnosis can be made based on history of exposure to plants listed in Table 3. A close clinical examination of the skin should be done with a magnifying glass or dermatoscope looking for residual trichomes or foreign bodies, which may continue to release irritant chemicals thus prolonging the reaction. If testing is desired, an open application test using the same method as above is recommended [5].

Treatment

Prevention is the ideal treatment as most reactions are self-limited. Patients who present with systemic symptoms or anaphylaxis should receive epinephrine, without delay. Other supportive therapies such as oxygen, albuterol, and intravenous steroids should be administered as needed [14].

Immunologic Contact Urticaria

Symptomatic treatment with topical, oral, or intravenous antihistamines such as diphenhydramine, hydroxyzine or cyproheptadine for up to two to five days is helpful for ICU [14]. In addition, local application of ice can help with subjective symptoms of burning and pain, when present. In patients presenting with systemic symptoms or anaphylaxis, epinephrine is the drug of choice. Patients with a history of severe urticaria, systemic symptoms, or anaphylaxis should carry a self-administrable epinephrine injection [14].

When work-related, improved occupational hygiene with the use of personal protective equipment is necessary. If attacks cannot be prevented and symptoms are significant, changing occupations may be necessary [18].

Non-immunologic Contact Urticaria

In patients with NICU, it is imperative to remove residual trichomes and foreign bodies, which can continue to release irritant chemicals for months [13]. In addition, patients should ensure there is not inadvertent, repeat exposure to trichomes by checking clothing and other accessories such as hats, backpacks, and shoes [14]. Several methods can be used to remove residual plant material from the skin such as applying warm wax, glue, plaster, or cellophane tape and then quickly removing to dislodge remaining appendages [36]. Topical or oral antihistamines such as diphenhydramine or hydroxyzine as well as topical pramoxine and oral non-steroidal anti-inflammatory medication can provide symptomatic relief.

Preventive Measures

Prevention strategies are neither novel nor foolproof and are mainly centered on avoidance.

The best prevention of ICU is allergen avoidance [4]. Those with mild symptoms such as localized urticaria, itching, burning, or erythema, may wear dry, clean, non-latex gloves when working with known urticants [3]. Those with a history of systemic involvement should avoid exposure at all costs and should seek emergency medical treatment at the first sign of systemic symptoms or anaphylaxis.

The best prevention of NICU also is avoidance. When avoidance is not possible, wearing protective clothing such as gloves, long sleeves, and long pants tucked into socks can prevent exposure. In general, all plants with trichomes or other sharp appendages should be avoided, especially if one is unfamiliar with the species. In addition, recognizing plants that cause NICU, especially *Urtica dioica* for those living in the United States, may help with avoidance (Figs. 3 and 4). If working, traveling, or exploring unfamiliar areas or areas known to have toxic plants, pack a small first-aid kit with 1st or 2nd generation H1-antihistamines, which may help lessen severity of symptoms following exposure.

References

1. Maurer M, Weller K, Bindslev-Jensen C, et al. Unmet clinical needs in chronic spontaneous urticaria. A GA^{2}LEN task force report. Allergy. 2011;66:317–30.
2. Lovell CR. Current topics in plant dermatitis. Semin Dermatol. 1996;15:113–21.
3. Amaro C, Goossens A. Immunological occupational contact urticaria and contact dermatitis from proteins: a review. Contact Dermatitis. 2008;58:67–75.
4. Ismail M, Maibach H. The clinical significance of immunological contact urticaria to processed grains. Indian J Dermatol Venereol Leprol. 2012;78:591–4.
5. Lahti A. Contact urticaria to plants. Clin Dermatol. 1986;4:127–36.
6. Konstantinou GN, Grattan CEH. Food contact hypersensitivity syndrome: the mucosal contact urticaria paradigm. Clin Exp Dermatol. 2008;33:383–9.
7. Muluk BN, Cingi C. Oral allergy syndrome. Am J Rhinol Allergy. 2018;32:27–30.
8. Kanerva L, Estlander T, Petman L, et al. Occupational allergic contact urticaria to yucca (*Yucca aloifolia*), weeping fig (*Ficus benhamina*) and spathe flower (*Spathiphyllum wallisii*). Allergy. 2001;56:1008–11.
9. Kiistala R, Makinen-Kiljunen S, Heikkinen K. Occupational allergic rhinitis and contact urticaria caused by bishop's weed (*Ammi majus*). Allergy. 1999;54:635–9.
10. Paulsen E, Andersen K. Lettuce contact allergy. Contact Dermat. 2015;74:67–75.
11. Piirila P, Kanerva L, Alanko K. Occupational IgE-mediated asthma, rhinoconjunctivitis and contact urticaria caused by Easter lily (*Lilium longiflorum*) and tulip. Allergy. 1998;54:273–7.
12. Oliver F, Amon EU, Breathnach A, et al. Contact urticaria due to the common stinging nettle (Urtica dioica)–histological, ultrastructural and pharmacological studies. Clin Exp Dermatol. 1991;16:1–7.
13. Maor D, Little M. Skin contact with a stinging tree requiring intensive care unit admission. Contact Dermat. 2017;77:325–51.
14. Freeman EE, Paul S, Shofner J, et al. Plant-induced dermatitis. In: Auerbach PS, Cushing TA, Stuart HN, editors. Auerbach's wilderness medicine. Elsevier; 2017. p. 1413–33.
15. Webster GL. Irritant plants in the spurge family (Euphorbiaceae). Clin Dermatol. 1986;4:36–45.
16. Lukacs J, Schliemann S, Elsner P. Occupational contact urticaria caused by food–a systemic clinical review. Contact Dermat. 2016;75:195–204.
17. Paulsen E, Sogaard J, Andersen KE. Occupational dermatitis in Danish gardeners and greenhouse workers (III). Contact Dermat. 1998;38:140–6.
18. Vester L, Thyssen J, Menne T. Consequences of occupational food-related hand dermatoses with a focus on protein contact dermatitis. Contact Dermat. 2012;67:328–33.
19. Cummings AJ, Olsen M. Mechanism of action of stinging nettles. Wilderness Environ Med. 2011;22:136–9.
20. Anderson BE, Miller CJ, Adams DR. Stinging nettle dermatitis. Am J Contact Dermatol. 2003;4:44–6.
21. USDA, NRCS. 2019. The PLANTS Database (http://plants.usda.goc, 9 April 2019). National Plant Data Team, Greensboro, NC 27401-4901 USA.
22. Ballmer-Weber BK, Hoffmann A, Wuthrich B, et al. Influence of food processing on the allergenicity of celery: DBPCFC with celery spice and cooked celery in patients with celery allergy. Allergy. 2002;57:228–35.
23. Bohle B, Zwolfer B, Heratizadeh A, et al. Cooking birch pollen-related food: divergent consequences of IgE- and T cell-mediated reactivity *in vitro* and *in vivo*. J Allergy Clin Immunol. 2006;118:242–9.

24. Sanchez MC, Hernandez M, Morena V, et al. Inmunologic contact urticaria caused by asparagus. Contact Dermat. 1997;37:181–2.
25. Weltfriend S, Kwangsukstith C, Maibach H. Contact urticaria from cucumber pickle and strawberry. Contact Dermat. 1995;32:173–4.
26. Barboud A, Poreux C, Penven E, Waton J. Occupational protein contact dermatitis. Eur J Dermatol. 2015;25:527–34.
27. Heloskoski E, Suojalehto H, Kuuliala O, et al. Occupational contact urticaria and protein contact dermatitis: causes and concomitant airway diseases. Contact Dermat. 2017;77:390–6.
28. Assarian Z, Nixon RL. Protein contact dermatitis caused by lime in a pastry chef. Contact Dermat. 2015;73:54–6.
29. Price A, Ramachandran S, Smith G, et al. Oral allergy syndrome (Pollen- Food Allergy Syndrome). Dermatitis. 2015;26(2):78–88.
30. Flores E, Cervera L, Sanz ML, et al. Plant food allergy in patients with pollinosis from the Mediterranean area. Int Arch Allergy Immunol. 2012;159(4):346–54.
31. Ballmer-Weber BK, Vieths S, Luttkopf D, et al. Celery allergy confirmed by double-blind, placebo-controlled food challenge: a clinical study in 32 subjects with a history of adverse reaction to celery root. J Allergy Clin Immunol. 2000;106:373–8.
32. Hansen KS, Ballmer-weber BK, Luttkopf D, et al. Roasted hazelnuts- allergenic activity evaluated by double-blind placebo-controlled food challenge. Allergy. 2003;58:132–8.
33. Fu HY, Chen JS, Chen FR, et al. Why do nettles sting? About stinging hairs looking simple but acting complex. Funct Plant Sci Biotechnol. 2007;1:45–55.
34. Ballero M, Piu G, Appendino G. Immediate urticaria to Euphorbiaceae. Allergy. 1999;54:91–2.
35. Schmitt C, Parola P, Haro L. Painful sting after exposure to dendrocnide sp: two case reports. Wilderness Environ Med. 2013;24:471–3.
36. Lindsey D, Lindsey WE. Cactus spine injuries. Am J Emerg Med. 1988;6:362–9.

Plant-Induced Irritant Contact Dermatitis

Reid A. Waldman and Jane M. Grant-Kels

Plants are a common and underreported cause of irritant contact dermatitis. Plant-induced irritant contact dermatitis is divided into two categories based on the type of 'irritant': (1) mechanical irritant contact dermatitis (MICD); and (2) chemical irritant contact dermatitis (CICD). While mechanical and chemical irritant contact dermatitis are distinct processes, they frequently present as an overlap condition termed mechano-irritant contact dermatitis where mechanical trauma facilitates the penetration of toxic chemicals. Common causes of mechanical and chemical irritant contact dermatitis due to plants, clinical manifestations of plant-induced irritant contact dermatitis, and complications of plant-induced irritant contact dermatitis are reviewed below.

Mechanical Irritant Contact Dermatitis (MICD)

Mechanical irritant contact dermatitis is defined as physical injury resulting from direct contact with a plant spinose structure. There are 7 distinct types of spinose structures that are implicated in the majority of cases of MICD. While each of these spinous structures induces mechanical irritant contact dermatitis by inducing physical trauma to the skin, they are differentiated from a botanical perspective based on the part of the plant from which they are derived. This differentiation is significant from a clinical standpoint as different types of spinose structures induce different types of damage to the skin. Table 1 lists common examples of each spinose structure.

R. A. Waldman (✉) · J. M. Grant-Kels
University of CT Health Center Dermatology Department, 21 South Road, Farmington, CT 06032, USA
e-mail: waldman@uchc.edu

J. M. Grant-Kels
e-mail: grant@uchc.edu

© Springer Nature Switzerland AG 2020
J. Trevino and A. Y-Y. Chen (eds.), *Dermatological Manual of Outdoor Hazards*,
https://doi.org/10.1007/978-3-030-37782-3_3

Table 1 Examples of plant spinosestructures

Scientific name	Common name
Trichomes and Bristles	
Cornus spp.	Dogwood
Ficus spp.	Figs
Urtica spp.	Nettles
Spines, Spinose Apical Processes, Spinose Teeth	
Agave spp.	Agave
Aloe spp.	Aloe
Opuntia spp.	Cacti
Thorns	
Citrus spp.	Citrus
Euphorbia milii	Crown of Thorns
Bougainvillea spp.	Bougainvillea
Prickles	
Rosa spp.	Roses
Rubus spp.	Blackberry

Trichomes and Bristles

Trichomes are known colloquially as hairs [1]. They are small, often microscopic, hair-like projections from plant epidermal tissue that serve principally to protect plants against small insect infestations but they may also serve to secrete certain plant products [1, 2]. While the term 'trichome' is frequently used interchangeably among non-botanists with the terms bristle, spine, thorn, and prickle, true trichomes are distinct from these other entities as trichomes are small and pliable. From an irritant contact dermatitis standpoint, the trichomes of the catchweed bedstraw (*Galium aparine*) are notable as they have a hook-like configuration that allows them to stick to clothing facilitating the development of irritant contact dermatitis in skin that comes in contact with affected clothing as well as in skin that comes into direct contact with the plant itself [3].

Bristles are a subtype of trichome that are distinguished from true trichomes based on the bristle's characteristic stiffness. Bristle and trichome are almost always used interchangeably within the dermatology literature despite their botanical differences. A notable example of a plant with bristles that cause irritant contact dermatitis is the wild comfrey (*Cynoglossum virginianum*) which is colloquially known as the "hound's tongue" because of the rough, tongue-like texture created by the plant's bristles [4].

Spines, Spinose Apical Processes, Spinose Teeth

Spines, spinose apical processes, spinose teeth, thorns, and prickles are all rigid, sharp projections that primarily serve to protect plants from larger herbivores such as birds, rabbits, and deer [5]. Spines are derived from plant leaves. While there are many types of spines, the spines of the *Opuntia species*, termed glochids, are of great importance to dermatologists as they are the cause of glochid dermatitis (also known as sabra dermatitis) [6]. The most commonly encountered *Opuntia* species is the prickly pear cactus which is harvested for its fruit and planted outside of buildings to serve as a physical deterrent to burglars (Fig. 1). Glochid dermatitis is important to recognize because management involves removing the numerous tiny glochids that lodge within a patient's skin [6].

Spinose apical processes are distinguished from spines based on their location. By definition, spinous apical processes are spines that are located on the apex of a leaf. The prototypical example of a spinose apical process is that of *aloe vera* which is frequently kept as a house plant and harvested for medicinal purposes [7].

Spinose teeth, also known as spinose leaf margin, are serrated spines that as the name suggests arise from a leaf's margin. Those present on Holly leaves (*ilex aquifolium*) are a frequently encountered example [7].

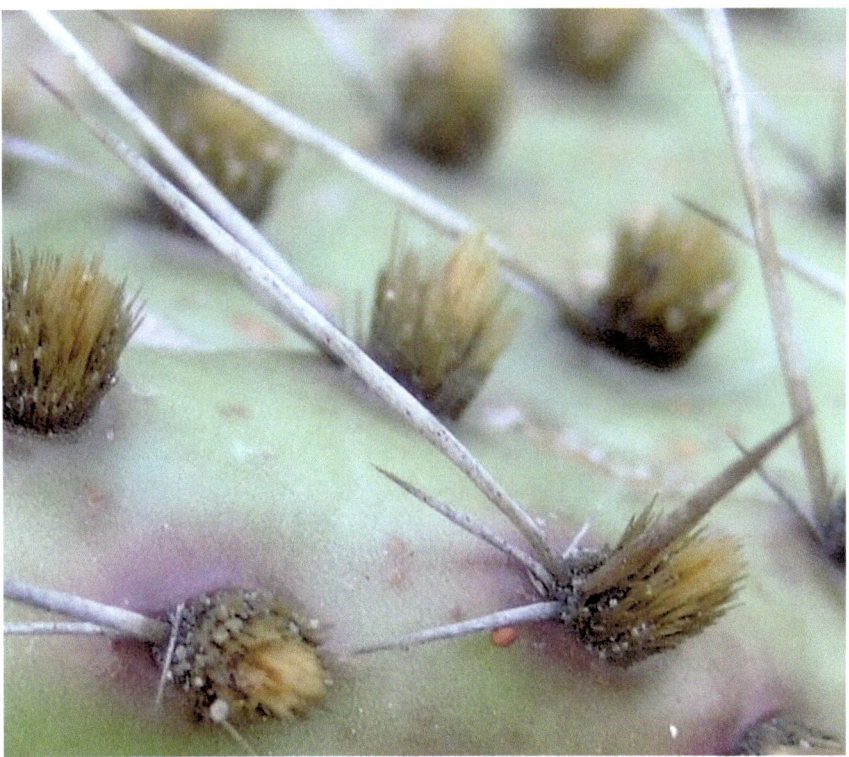

Fig. 1 Spines and glochids of a Prickly Pear Cactus (Courtesy Creative Commons, photograph by Succu zoom by RoRo). https://commons.wikimedia.org/wiki/File:Succu_Opuntia_howeyi_02_detail_-_spines_and_glochids.jpg

Thorns

Thorns are distinguished from spines and their aforementioned subtypes both in derivation and morphology. Thorns arise from plant shoots and therefore are morphologically distinct because they can branch and may possess leaves [8]. Importantly, many plants that are described in the vernacular as having thorns (e.g. *rose* species) actually have prickles. In contradistinction, *citrus* species have true thorns (Fig. 2) [9].

Prickles

Prickles arise from the plant epidermis and cortex and are distinct from spines and thorns as they lack a vascular bundle [8]. They are also distinct from trichomes and bristles because they are derived from both the cortex, the layer between the epidermis and the vascular bundle, and the epidermis, the outermost layer of cells of a plant, and they are more rigid [7, 10]. The prototypical example of a plant with prickles is the *rosa* species (Fig. 3).

Wood Splinter

Wood splinters are the most common foreign bodies in the skin. Wood splinters can be acquired either through contact with live plants or contact with wood products such as mulch that is placed around plants.

Complications of Mechanical Irritant Contact Dermatitis

Mechanical irritant contact dermatitis can be complicated by the development of a foreign body granuloma to retained plant matter and by the development of an infection due to direct inoculation of a microbe by the spinose process.

Granuloma Formation

Plant matter that is traumatically inoculated into the skin is a common cause of foreign body granuloma [11]. Clinically, plant matter protruding from the skin may or may not be identified and the exact clinical presentation varies based on duration and depth of implantation. When the diagnosis is not readily apparent and biopsy is performed, histopathologic examination reveals a foreign body

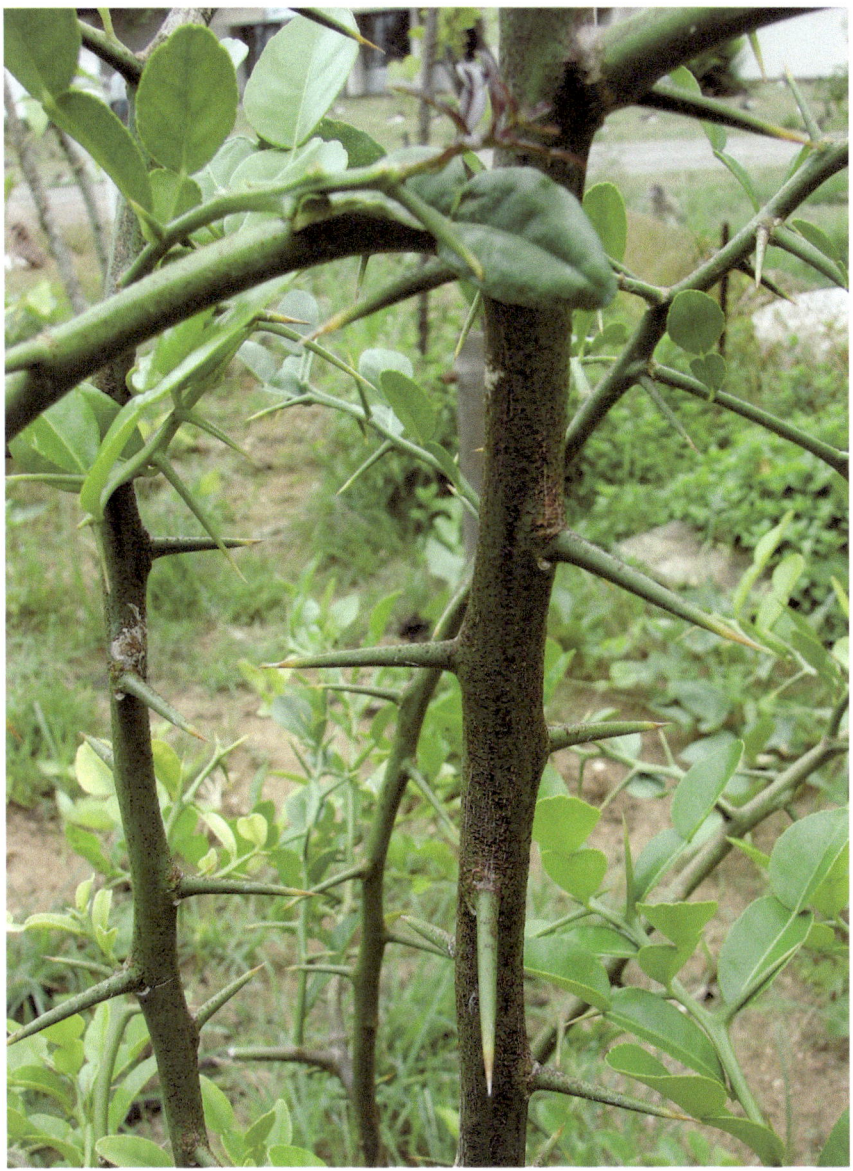

Fig. 2 Thorns of the Citrus Hystrix **(Courtesy Creative Commons, photograph by Forest and Kim Starr).** https://commons.wikimedia.org/wiki/File:Starr-080610-8293-Citrus_hystrix-thorns-Community_Garden_Sand_Island-Midway_Atoll_(24893012816).jpg

granuloma containing PAS-positive, birefringent material [11]. Some plant materials such as wood splinters and 'glochids' have characteristic features on histopathologic examination [11–13]. Foreign body granulomas must be differentiated from infection as the two may co-exist or mimic one another and they require

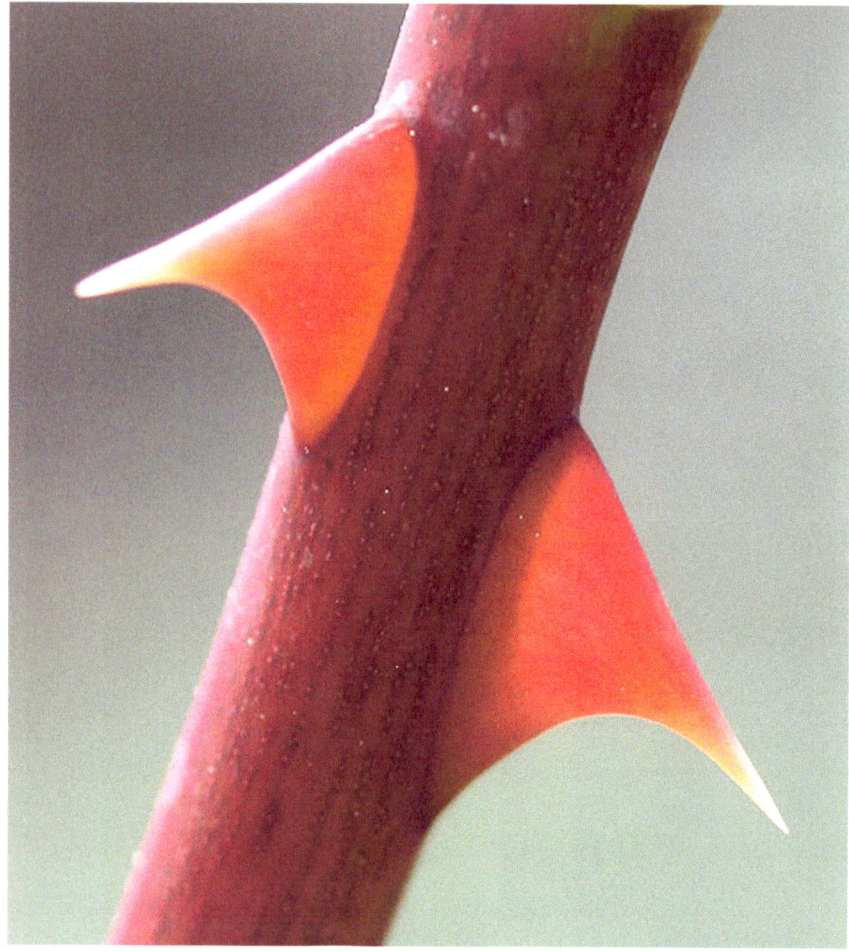

Fig. 3 Rose prickles (Courtesy Creative Commons, Photographed by John Desjarlais). https://commons.wikimedia.org/wiki/File:Rose_prickle.jpg

different management strategies. Management of plant material-induced foreign body granulomas requires the removal of the foreign material as chronically retained plant material can serve as a nidus for infection and can induce inflammatory damage to the underlying bone and joints [14].

Infection

Cutaneous trauma induced by plant material can inoculate bacteria and fungi into the skin resulting in infection. The prototype for this type of infection is *Sporothrix schenkii*, the dimorphous fungus responsible for sporotrichosis, which is frequently inoculated by traumatic contact with *rose* prickles [15]. Through similar mechanisms of seeding, many other bacteria and fungi can cause mechanical irritant contact dermatitis -related infections.

Chemical Irritant Contact Dermatitis

Some plants produce chemicals which are most commonly excreted within their sap that can cause irritant contact dermatitis when they contact the skin. These chemicals can be subdivided into several overarching classes that are produced by a variety of different plant species (Table 2).

Alkaloids

Alkaloids are nitrogen-containing bases. More than 12,000 types of alkaloids have been identified and at least 20% of flowering plants produce alkaloids [16]. Alkaloids can be present in the leaves, bark, and roots of plants [16]. Commonly

Table 2 Examples of plants that cause chemical ICD

Scientific name	Common name
Alkaloids	
Atropa belladonna	Belladonna or Deadly Nightshade
Narcissus spp.	Daffodil
Nicotiana spp.	Tobacco
Bromelain	
Ananas comosus	Pineapple
Calcium Oxalate	
Narcissus spp.	Daffodil
Dieffenbachia spp.	Dumb Cane
Philodendron spp.	Philodendron
Diterpene Esters	
Euphorbia pulcherrima	Poinsettia
Croton tiglium	Purging Croton
Euphorbia peplus	Milkweed
Isothiocyanates	
Eutrema japonicum	Wasabi
Armoracia rusticana	Horseradish
Brassica spp.	Mustard
Juglone	
Juglone spp.	Walnut
Protoanemonin	
Ranunculus spp.	Buttercups

encountered alkaloids include nicotine, morphine, strychnine, cocaine, and atropine [16]. The alkaloid that is most commonly implicated in plant chemical irritant contact dermatitis and that is also frequently employed therapeutically within dermatology is capsaicin (8-methyl-N-vanillyl-6-nonenamide) [17]. Capsaicin is produced by the *Solanaceae* family which includes many types of chili peppers (Fig. 4) [17]. The mechanism of capsaicin-induced irritant contact dermatitis is unique in that it does not directly result in tissue damage like other chemical irritants. Instead, it is an agonist of the vanilloid receptor subtype 1 [18]. This agonism triggers neuron activation which results in the sensation of heat. A unique clinical phenotype associated with cutaneous exposure to capsaicin is called the "Hunan Hand" which occurs from prolonged exposure of the hands to chili peppers while cooking [17]. This condition earned its appellation as it was initially described in an individual cooking a traditional Hunan meal with dried red chili peppers (*Capsicum japonicum*). Not all alkaloids behave like capsaicin. Many alkaloids do not cause mechanical irritant contact dermatitis and others can only cause dermatitis in the setting of a simultaneous mechanical irritant contact dermatitis (i.e. mechano-irritant contact dermatitis).

Bromelain

Bromelain is a family of sulfhydryl proteolytic enzymes produced by pineapples (*Ananas comosus*, Fig. 5). Bromelain is a frequent cause of chemical irritant contact dermatitis and stomatitis [19]. It less frequently can also cause an allergic contact dermatitis [19]. It is used in the culinary industry as a meat tenderizer and also used in folk medicine as a digestion aid, blood thinner, as well as for wound debridement [20].

Calcium Oxalate

Calcium oxalate is a calcium salt that frequently forms needle-shaped crystals called raphides within plants [21]. These raphides cause penetrative injury to tissue they come into contact with and then facilitate the penetration of other plant toxins and chemical irritants. Calcium oxalate is ubiquitous among plants. Commonly encountered plants with high concentrations of calcium oxalate include daffodils (*Narcissus*), tulips (*Tulipa*, Fig. 6), and dumb cane (*Dieffenbachia*) [7]. In each of these plants, calcium oxalate raphides facilitate penetration of many other toxins and chemical irritants.

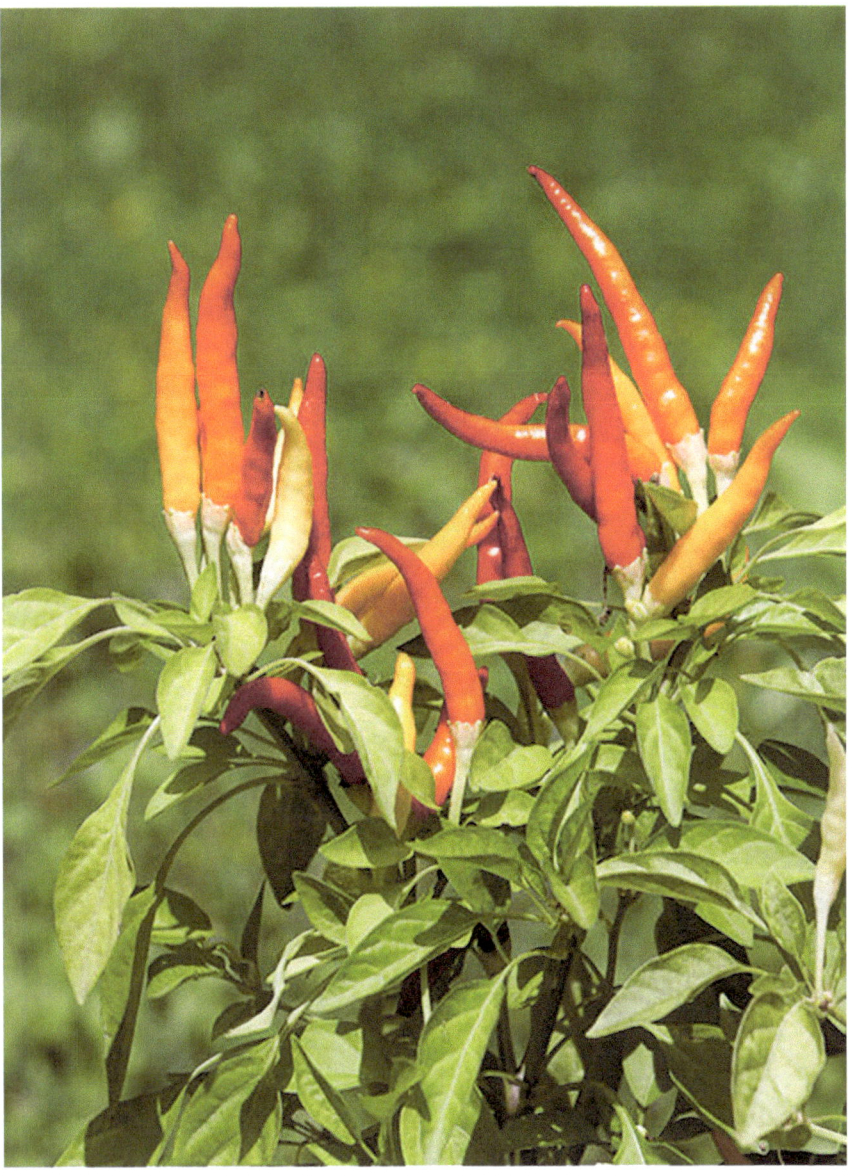

Fig. 4 Capsicum Anuum var. Fiesta (Courtesy Creative Commons, Photographed by PierreS-elim). https://commons.wikimedia.org/wiki/File:Capsicum_annuum_var._Fiesta_-_MHNT.jpg

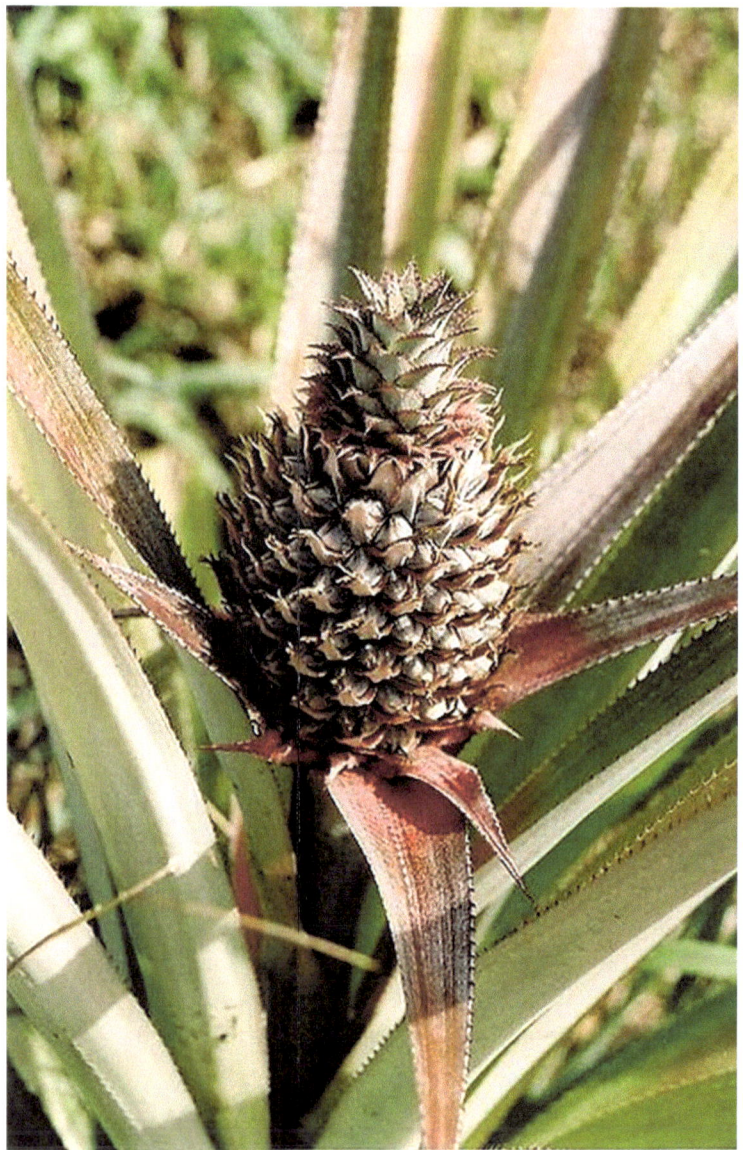

Fig. 5 Pineapple plant (Courtesy Creative Commons, Photographed by Nick Lott). https://commons.wikimedia.org/wiki/File:Young_Pineapple.jpg

Diterpene Esters

Diterpene esters are a group of voracious irritants that are most commonly produced by members of the "spurge" family [22]. The *Euphorbiaceae* family earned the colloquial appellation "spurge" because ingestion of these plants results

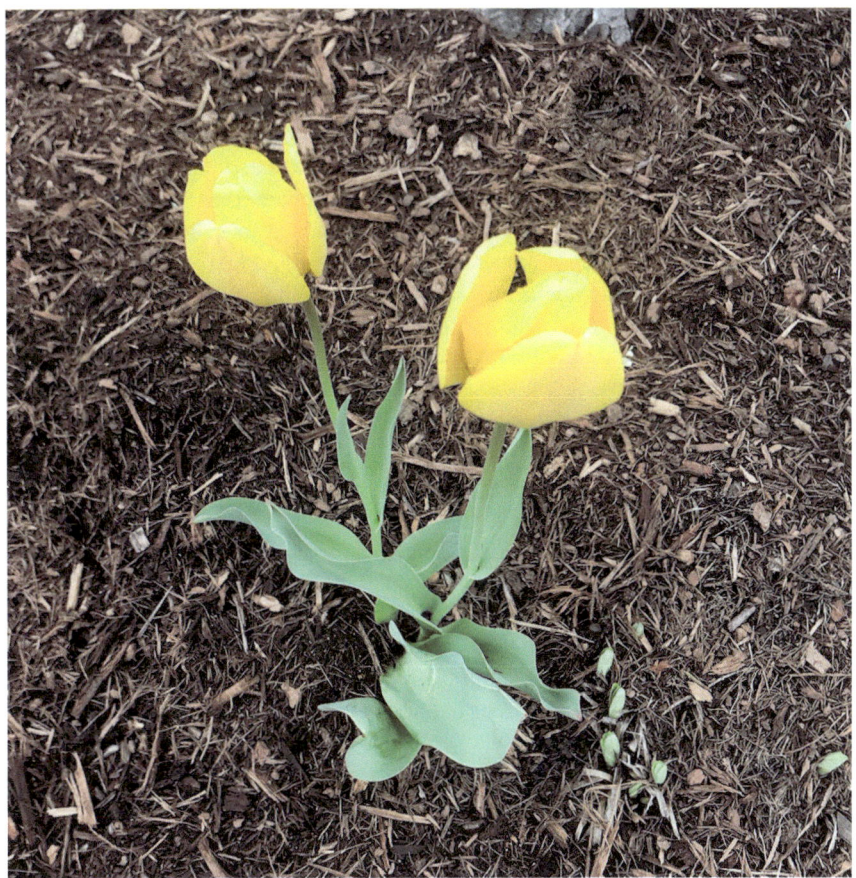

Fig. 6 Tulip (Courtesy of Reid Waldman, MD and Kelley Sharp, BSN)

in a purge of vomiting and diarrhea. Diterpene esters can be subclassified into daphnane, lathyrane, tigliane, and ingenane varieties based on structure. The most dermatologically relevant diterpene esters are ingenol mebutate and phorbol esters [22]. A formulation of ingenol mebutate is commercially available for treatment of actinic keratoses under the trade name of Picato®; whereas, croton oil, a type of phorbol ester, is the most important ingredient in the Baker-Gordon chemical peel.

From an irritant contact dermatitis perspective, diterpene esters are significant because: (1) they are found in the sap of thousands of diverse plants present all over the world; (2) the irritant contact dermatitis caused by diterpene esters is often very severe and can mimic allergic contact dermatitis caused by *Toxicodendron* species; and (3) if ingested, diterpene esters can cause severe vomiting and diarrhea [22].

Isothiocyanates

Isothiocyanates are plant secondary products that are created from hydrolysis of plant glucosinolates [23]. Isothiocyanates are almost exclusively found in plants belonging to *Brassicaceae*, *Capparaceae* and *Caricacea* families [23]. Plants that produce isothiocyanates can be divided into cruciferous vegetables such as cauliflower and bok choy and into plants that produce mustard oils (allyl isothiocyanate) such as mustard, horseradish, and wasabi. Most contact with plants that produce isothiocyanates occurs among chefs. The irritant contact dermatitis created by isothiocyanates is mild and short-lived much like the spicy sensation experienced by diners that consume them. Isothiocyanates also cause conjunctival injection and irritation which is why allyl isothiocyanate was adapted into mustard gas for use as a chemical weapon.

Juglone

Juglone is a naphthoquinone produced by the walnut tree (*Juglans regia*). It is present in the nuts, husks, and bark of the tree [24]. Juglone has been recognized as an important product of the walnut tree for centuries as it is toxic to plants grown in the vicinity of walnut trees and it can be used as a skin and hair dye [24]. Juglone is an interesting cause of chemical irritant contact dermatitis because it hyperpigments the skin it comes in contact with through a mechanism similar to henna. Henna may cause a juglone-induced dermatitis that can be misdiagnosed as furocoumarin-induced phytophotodermatitis [25, 26].

Protoanemonin

Protoanemonin is a DNA polymerase inhibitor produced by all members of the Buttercup (*Ranunculus*) family [27, 28]. It is a degradation product of the glucoside ranunculin which is generated when members of the buttercup family are crushed or otherwise injured. Most reported cases of protoanemonin-induced irritant contact dermatitis occur in the Middle East where certain groups use buttercup flowers as traditional herbal remedies for arthritis, abscesses, and a number of other conditions [29]. The irritant contact dermatitis caused by protoanemonin is severe and results from disruption of epidermal disulfide bonds which explains why protoanemonin-induced dermatitis frequently presents with epidermal bullae [27].

Conclusion

Plants are a common cause of irritant contact dermatitis that can cause diverse presentations depending on the implicated irritant. Given the frequency of plant-induced irritant contact dermatitis, dermatologists should be familiar with common and novel causes of plant-induced ICD. By correctly identifying the cause of a patient's contact dermatitis, dermatologists can help the patient develop practical irritant avoidance strategies and prevent repeated and worsening bouts of plant-induced irritant contact dermatitis. Dermatologists can also prescribe topical corticosteroids and tailor implementation of protective measures including pre-exposure application of barrier creams and use of protective clothing (e.g. gloves) in cases where exposure is unavoidable.

References

1. Liu H, Liu S, Jiao J, Lu TJ, Xu F. Trichomes as a natural biophysical barrier for plants and their bioinspired applications. Soft Matter. 2017;13(30):5096–106.
2. Huchelmann A, Boutry M, Hachez C. Plant Glandular Trichomes: Natural Cell Factories of High Biotechnological Interest. Plant Physiol. 2017;175(1):6–22.
3. Bowling AJ, Maxwell HB, Vaughn KC. Unusual trichome structure and composition in mericarps of catchweed bedstraw (Galium aparine). Protoplasma. 2008;233(3–4):223–30.
4. Modi GM, Doherty CB, Katta R, Orengo IF. Irritant contact dermatitis from plants. Dermat Contact Atopic Occup Drug. 2009;20(2):63–78.
5. Kariyat RR, Hardison SB, De Moraes CM, Mescher MC. Plant spines deter herbivory by restricting caterpillar movement. Biol Lett [Internet]. 2017 May [cited 2019 Apr 21];13(5). https://www.ncbi.nlm.nih.gov/pmc/articles/PMC5454246/.
6. Suárez A, Freeman S, Puls L, Dellavalle R. Unusual presentation of cactus spines in the flank of an elderly man: a case report. J Med Case Rep. 2010;25(4):152.
7. Otang WM, Grierson DS, Afolayan AJ. A survey of plants responsible for causing irritant contact dermatitis in the Amathole district, Eastern Cape. South Africa J Ethnopharmacol. 2014;18(157):274–84.
8. Plant Systematics—2nd Edition [Internet]. [cited 2019 Apr 21]. https://www.elsevier.com/books/plant-systematics/simpson/978-0-08-092208-9.
9. Roth LM, Levin EH, Schwartz AH, Roth DJ. Phytophotodermatitis due to puncture from lime tree thorn. South Med J. 2007;100(5):544–5.
10. Botany online: Dermal Tissues—Cross-Section—Prickle—Rose [Internet]. 2008 [cited 2019 Apr 21]. https://web.archive.org/web/20080430190522/, http://www.biologie.uni-hamburg.de/b-online/e05/stachel.htm.
11. Butler WP. Plant thorn granuloma. Mil Med. 1995;160(1):39.
12. Whiting DA, Bristow JH. Dermatitis and keratoconjunctivitis caused by a prickly pear (Opuntia microdasys). South Afr Med J Suid-Afr Tydskr Vir Geneeskd. 1975;49(35):1445–8.
13. Requena L, Cerroni L, Kutzner H. Histopathologic patterns associated with external agents. Dermatol Clin. 2012;30(4):731–48, vii.
14. Schreiber MM, Shapiro SI, Berry CZ. Cactus granulomas of the skin: an allergic phenomenon. Arch Dermatol. 1971;104(4):374–9.
15. Kieselova K, Santiago F, Henrique M. Rose thorn injury. BMJ Case Rep. 2017;22

16. Richard T, Temsamani H, Cantos-Villar E, Monti J-P. Chapter Two—Application of LC–MS and LC–NMR techniques for secondary metabolite identification. In: Rolin D, editor. Advances in botanical research [Internet]. Academic Press; 2013 [cited 2019 Apr 21]. p. 67–98. (Metabolomics Coming of Age with its Technological Diversity; vol. 67). http://www.sciencedirect.com/science/article/pii/B9780123979223000022.

17. Williams SR, Clark RF, Dunford JV. Contact dermatitis associated with capsaicin: Hunan hand syndrome. Ann Emerg Med. 1995;25(5):713–5.

18. Szallasi A, Blumberg PM. Vanilloid (Capsaicin) receptors and mechanisms. Pharmacol Rev. 1999;51(2):159–212.

19. Raison-Peyron N, Roulet A, Guillot B, Guilhou JJ. Bromelain: an unusual cause of allergic contact cheilitis. Contact Dermat. 2003;49(4):218–9.

20. Hirche C, Citterio A, Hoeksema H, Koller J, Lehner M, Martinez JR, et al. Eschar removal by bromelain based enzymatic debridement (Nexobrid®) in burns: an European consensus. Burns J Int Soc Burn Inj. 2017;43(8):1640–53.

21. Raman V, Horner HT, Khan IA. New and unusual forms of calcium oxalate raphide crystals in the plant kingdom. J Plant Res. 2014;127(6):721–30.

22. Huerth KA, Hawkes JE, Meyer LJ, Powell DL. The scourge of the spurge family—an imitator of Rhus dermatitis. Dermat Contact Atopic Occup Drug. 2016;27(6):372–81.

23. Milanesi N, Gola M. Irritant contact dermatitis caused by Savoy cabbage. Contact Dermat. 2016;74(1):60–1.

24. Talcott P. Chapter 21—Toxicologic problems. In: Reed SM, Bayly WM, Sellon DC, editors. Equine internal medicine, 4h ed. [Internet]. W.B. Saunders; 2018 [cited 2019 Apr 21]. p. 1460–512. http://www.sciencedirect.com/science/article/pii/B9780323443296000218.

25. Bonamonte D, Foti C, Angelini G. Hyperpigmentation and contact dermatitis due to *Juglans regia*. Contact Dermat. 2001;44(2):101–2.

26. Neri I, Bianchi F, Giacomini F, Patrizi A. Acute irritant contact dermatitis due to *Juglans regia*. Contact Dermat. 2006;55(1):62–3.

27. Calka O, Omer C, Akdeniz N, Necmettin A, Özkol HU, Ozkol Hatice U, et al. Irritant contact dermatitis caused by Ranunculus kotschyi Boiss in 6 cases. Contact Dermatitis. 2011;64(3):174–6.

28. Metin A, Calka O, Behçet L, Yildirim E. Phytodermatitis from *Ranunculus damascenus*. Contact Dermat. 2001;44(3):183.

29. Ozkol HU, Calka O, Akdeniz N, Pinar SM. Phytodermatitis in eastern Turkey: a retrospective, observational study. Dermat Contact Atopic Occup Drug. 2014;25(3):140–6.

Phytophotodermatitis

Daniel A. Nguyen, Muneeza K. Muhammad and Grace L. Lee

Abbreviations

PUVA   Psoralen and Ultraviolet A Radiation
ROS   Reactive Oxygen Species
UVA   Ultraviolet A Radiation

Background/Introduction

Certain plant compounds may be toxic via direct human skin contact, while others may become phototoxic when combined with light. Dr. Robert Klaber originally coined the term "phytophotodermatitis" in a 1942 publication of the British Journal of Dermatology and Syphilis. Dr. Klaber suggested this term to describe the phenomenon of human skin eruptions produced by photosensitizing plants and their extracts upon exposure to sunlight [1].

Phytophotodermatitis may have only recently been coined as a term, but historical characterizations have been described as far back as 2000 B.C. in Egypt [2]. Egyptians used the Apiaceae plant family species *Ammi majus*, also known as false Bishop's Weed, to treat vitiligo [2, 3]. Apiaceae (formerly known as Umbelliferae) is among the commonly implicated plant families along with Rutaceae and

D. A. Nguyen
Medical City Weatherford, Weatherford, TX 76086, USA
e-mail: daniel.nguyen2@medicalcityhealth.com

M. K. Muhammad · G. L. Lee (✉)
Baylor College of Medicine Department of Dermatology, Houston, TX 77030, USA
e-mail: gllee@texaschildrens.org

G. L. Lee
Texas Children's Hospital Pediatric Dermatology, Houston, TX 77030, USA

© Springer Nature Switzerland AG 2020
J. Trevino and A. Y-Y. Chen (eds.), *Dermatological Manual of Outdoor Hazards*,
https://doi.org/10.1007/978-3-030-37782-3_4

Moraceae. A sizable portion of phytophotodermatitis literature is found in dermatological publications, but efforts have been made to raise awareness across multidisciplinary teams including emergency and burn personnel [4]. Even the media has drawn attention to devastating plant effects with captivating articles such as the BBC's report on 'Giant hogweed 'UK's most dangerous plant' [4, 5].

Classification/Description of Plants Discussed

Photosensitizer

The phototoxic plants share common constituents that react with light. The prototypical photosensitizing compound is the furocoumarin, which combines a furan ring with coumarin [3]. Depending on the furan position, furocoumarins can be further classified into linear furocoumarins (e.g. psoralen) or angular furocoumarins (e.g. angelicin) [3]. Psoralen (specifically 8-methoxypsoralen) is the substance commonly recognized as the photosensitizing agent used in a photodynamic therapy known as PUVA (psoralen and UVA) [4].

Naturally, the furocoumarins are thought to provide protection against predators, such as fungus or herbivores [4, 6–8]. The psoralens in celery have shown to be increased when actively infected with fungus [6, 9]. Handlers of increased quantities of celery have reported skin eruptions [6, 9].

The detrimental effects of phytophotodermatitis are Type I or Type II phototoxic reactions leading to DNA damage or reactive oxygen species (ROS), respectively [4, 7]. In Type I reactions, there is covalent bonding of monofunctional adducts and bifunctional interstrand cross-links between the furan ring on the furocoumarin and pyrimidine bases of nuclear DNA [7, 10, 11]. In Type II reactions, ROS causes oxidative damage by interacting with proteins, DNA, and/or lipids [10]. Both reaction types are both triggered by UVA radiation (320–400 nm), with both natural (i.e. sun) or artificial (i.e. tanning salons) sources implicated [3, 4, 11, 12]. These phototoxic reactions lead to mutations, cell membrane damage, inflammation, and cell death [3, 10, 11, 13].

Apiaceae

Apiaceae (Umbelliferae) may be the most well-known phototoxic plant family. Apiaceae are found worldwide with many species containing phototoxic furocoumarins [3, 10, 14]. This family of plants is particularly recognized for its umbel structure design [3, 14]. Like an umbrella, the structure is illustrated by a cluster of flowers with its stalks, or pedicels, all originating from a common center point [3, 14]. A number of Apiaceae are recognizable vegetables such as celery, parsley, parsnip, carrot, fennel, and dill. [3, 10, 14]. Table 1 provides a detailed list of phototoxic plants, including relevant Apiaceae plants.

Table 1 Detailed list of phototoxic plants

Family	Species	Common name
Apiaceae	*Amni majus*	Queen Anne's lace, False Bishop's weed
Apiaceae	*Anethum graveolens*	Dill
Apiaceae	*Angelica archangelica*	Angelica
Apiaceae	*Angelica sylvestris*	Wild angelica
Apiaceae	*Anthriscus sylvestris*	Cow parsley, wild chervil
Apiaceae	*Apium graveolens*	Celery
Apiaceae	*Chaerophyllum macropodum* **Boiss**	
Apiaceae	*Daucus carota*	Carrot
Apiaceae	*Ferula orientalis*	
Apiaceae	*Foeniculum vulgare*	Fennel
Apiaceae	*Heracleum lanatum*	Cow parsnip
Apiaceae	*Heracleum mantegazzianum*	Giant hogweed
Apiaceae	*Heracleum persicum*	Persian hogweed, golpar
Apiaceae	*Heracleum sosnowskyi*	Sosnowskyi's hogweed
Apiaceae	*Heracleum sphondylium*	Cow parsnip, hogweed, cow parsley
Apiaceae	*Notobubon galbanum*	Blister bush, hog's fennel
Apiaceae	*Pastinaca sativa*	Parsnip
Apiaceae	*Petroselinum crispum*	Parsley
Apiaceae	*Peucedanum paniculatum* **Loisel**	
Apiaceae	*Pimpinella anisum*	Anise
Rutaceae	*Citrus aurantifolia*	Lime
Rutaceae	*Citrus aurantium*	Bitter orange
Rutaceae	*Citrus bergamia*	Bergamot orange
Rutaceae	*Citrus latifolia*	Persian limes, Tahiti limes, Bearss limes
Rutaceae	*Citrus limetta*	Sweet lemon
Rutaceae	*Citrus limon*	Lemon
Rutaceae	*Citrus maxima*	Zabon, pomelo
Rutaceae	*Citrus medica*	Citron
Rutaceae	*Citrus paradisi*	Grapefruit
Rutaceae	*Citrus sinensis*	Sweet orange
Rutaceae	*Dictamnus albus*	Burning bush, dittany, gas plant, fraxinella
Rutaceae	*Pelea anisata*	Mokihana
Rutaceae	*Ptelea crenulata*	California hoptree
Rutaceae	*Ptelea trifoliata*	Water ash
Rutaceae	*Rhadinothamnus anceps*	Blister bush
Rutaceae	*Ruta graveolens*	Common rue
Moraceae	*Ficus carica*	Common Fig
Moraceae	*Ficus pumila*	Creeping Fig

(continued)

Table 1 (continued)

Family	Species	Common name
Asteraceae	*Echinops exaltus*	Globe thistle
Asteraceae	*Tagetes patula*	French marigold
Berberidaceae	*Mahonia aquifolium*	Oregon grape
Chenopodiaceae	*Chenopodium album*	Lamb's quarters, melde, white goosefoot
Hypericaceae	*Hypericum perfoliatum*	
Hypericaceae	*Hypericum perforatum*	St. John's wort
Hypericaceae	*Hypericum tetrapterum*	St. Peter's wort
Leguminosae	*Cicer arietinum*	Chick Peas
Leguminosae	*Glycine max*	Soy beans
Leguminosae	*Myroxylon balsamum*	Balsam of Peru
Leguminosae	*Pisum sativum*	Pea
Leguminosae	*Psoralea corylifolia*	Bavchi, Scurf pea
Plantaginaceae	*Plantago lanceolata*	Ribwort plantain, narrowleaf plantain, English plantain, ribleaf, lamb's tongue
Polygonaceae	*Fagopyrum esculentum*	Buckwheat
Ranunculaceae	*Hydrastis canadensis*	Goldenseal
Ranunculaceae	*Ranunculus* sp.	Various
Rubiaceae	*Coffea arabica*	Coffee
Rubiaceae	*Gardenia* sp.	Various
Solanaceae	*Capsicum annuum*	Chili pepper

For an extensive list, please see texts by Murray, and Sarker and Nahar [72–77]

In a 2015 Polish study, Rzymski et al. surveyed forest employees about the Apiaceae *Heracleum sosnowskyi* and *Heracleum mantegazzianum*, commonly referred to as giant hogweeds [11]. The native Eurasian plants spread during the 20th century and became an invasive threat to central European biodiversity [15]. The Polish study revealed a general awareness of the plants, but a lack of plant management practice knowledge. These plants serve as a stark reminder of our dynamic environments and the importance of updating our knowledge base [11, 15]. An and Ozturk conducted a prospective study from Turkey identifying phytophotodermatitis implicating *Heracleum persicum*, *Ferula orientalis*, and *Chaerophyllum macropodum* Boiss, with the latter two being the first time described in the literature [16]. A report from France in 2018 claimed to be the first phytophotodermatitis case implicating native plant *Peucedanum paniculatum* Loisel [17]. Two carrot phytophotodermatitis cases have been reported—one from carrot extract containing sunscreen in 2018 and the other from a carrot decoction for wet compresses in 2011 [18, 19].

Rutaceae

Rutaceae is another common plant family that is widely known for its citrus fruits including lime, lemon, orange, grapefruit and pomelo [3, 20]. The often dubbed "other lime disease" involving the many citrus fruits has become some of the most widely reported phytophotodermatitis cases in recent times [21–33]. This is likely attributed to their increased use during travels, celebrations, and to their use with alcoholic beverages (mojitos, sangrias, and margaritas) [21–33]. The phototoxic oils are often found in the outermost layer of the peel, which have been used as zest in cooking [14]. Prospective study of orange and bergamot oil testing on mouse fibroblast cells demonstrated phototoxic levels despite low concentrations [34].

Other well-known Rutaceae include the common rue (*Ruta graveolens*) and its association with strimmer (i.e. string trimmer) dermatitis. With any common domestic vegetation, children who play outside may be exposed [35]. Rue is used as an herbal medicine for sprains, rheumatic pains, bruises, burns, and as an anti-parasitic agent and insect repellant [35–37].

The aromatic gas plant (*Dictamnus albus*) is another popular member of the Rutaceae family. This bush can briefly be ignited without harm and is thought to be the origin for the "burning bush of Moses" in the Bible [3, 10, 14]. Another Rutaceae member, mokihana (*Pelea anisata*), has been used in leis of Hawaii thus causing outbreaks around the neck [3, 10, 14]. Table 1 provides a detailed list of phototoxic Rutaceae plants.

Moraceae

Moraceae, or the Mulberry family, contains the fig tree (*Ficus caricu*), perhaps its most well-known phototoxic plant. While fig has been used on vitiligo for millennia, recent case reports continue to show fig to be an underrecognized cause of phytophotodermatitis outbreaks [3, 7, 10, 14, 38, 39]. The highest concentrations of furocoumarins are in the fig leaves and the shoot sap, particularly during spring or summer [40].

Another fig species which was implicated in its first case of phytophotodermatitis in 2012 is *Ficus pumila*, or creeping fig [41]. The ornamental plant was trimmed with a chainsaw and caused an eruption to a man's exposed arms and forehead, confirmed with a positive photopatch test [41]. Table 1 provides a detailed list of phototoxic Moraceae plants.

Other Families

Plant species from other plant families have been reported to induce phototoxic reactions in the literature. The Hypericaceae family's best-known phototoxic plant may be *Hypericum perforatum* or St. John's Wort. This popular herbal medicine often used for depression can cause phototoxic reactions in animals and humans [3, 42, 43]. A recent comparative study looked at 11 other species from the Hypericum family and identified, *H. perforatum*, *H. perfoliatum*, and *H. tetrapterum* as being phototoxic with an associated increase in naphthodianthrone compounds (photosensitizer) [44]. Another ancient remedy that again utilized the phototoxic effects of plants to treat vitiligo was *Psoralea corylifoli* of the Leguminosae (or Fabaceae) family [3, 10, 14, 45]. A case report describes a 30-year-old man with erythema, itching, blistering, and hyperpigmentation after receiving infusions of *P. corylifolii* and being exposed to the sun [46]. Two other Turkish studies noted two newly-reported plants producing phytophotodermatitis [47, 48]. *Chenopodium album* (Chenopodiaceae family) produced phototoxic reactions in 12 of 30 patients from a retrospective observational study [48]. Two cases of phytophotodermatitis have been reported from consumption of *Plantago lanceolata* (Plantaginaceae family) [47]. Table 1 provides a detailed list of phototoxic plants.

Epidemiology of Health Conditions Caused by the Plants

The epidemiology of phytophotodermatitis is quite variable and largely dependent on the plants implicated. Phytophotodermatitis can occur in any part of the world where vegetation exists. Specific phototoxic plants can be native to a local area, but invasive plants (e.g. giant hogweed) have spread across the globe and caused large economic impacts [11, 15, 49, 50].

Few studies look specifically at phytophotodermatitis epidemiology in general, but some studies investigate certain epidemiologic aspects or particular plants. Rzymski et al. in the Polish study investigated giant hogweeds for their distribution, awareness, and risk to forest employees [11]. Of the 1,563 employees, >50% reported that the plants were in their working area, >95% were aware of the plants, and >20% had been exposed the plant at least once in their life [11]. In An and Ozturk's prospective study at various Turkish hospitals and clinics, the frequency of phytophotodermatitis was 20.5% (7) of 34 phytodermatitis (includes phytophotodermatitis, irritant contact dermatitis, and allergic contact dermatitis) patients [16]. Baseline demographics showed more men were affected (67.6%) with a mean age of 31.9 years (range 9–67 years) and lesions primarily located on the arms and legs [16]. A two and a half year retrospective Croatian study found 16 phytophotodermatitis cases occurring more commonly in women (62.5%) with a mean age 31.9 (range 6–62 years) and 25% due to unknown plants. 31.3% occurred in the pediatric population in this study [51]. The limited cases of reported phytophotodermatitis may be the result of an asymptomatic manifestation that results in hyperpigmentation only [12].

Various factors can influence phytophotodermatitis. Within geographic locations, plant growth can vary from natural habitats such as forest or streams to domestic areas of neighborhoods and roads. Timing of plant growth may vary as plants can be perennial (e.g. *Heracleum mantegazzianum*) or seasonal (e.g. limes and their use in beverages). Seasons have also been known to affect furocoumarin concentrations [52].

Different populations have variable levels of risk. Professional workers involved in agriculture, gardening/yard work, lumberjacks, forestry, outdoor parks, or food handlers all have an increased occupational risk of contact with plants. Children may be at increased risk due to recreational activities outside or due to the attractive features of specific plants. Individual behaviors can play a large role in exposure risk as well. Application of herbal medications has been linked to a number of cases [3, 7, 10, 36, 46, 53, 54]. People who tan are more likely to have sun exposure and an increased risk or extent of damage if previously exposed to phototoxic plants. Even certain diets can influence behavior and lead to rare oral absorption and subsequent phytophotodermatitis, as exemplified by a celery soup diet resulting in a phototoxic rash [55]. Those who celebrate with alcoholic beverages that include citrus fruit, or those in the tourism service industry (bartenders), may have additional plant toxin and sunlight exposure, increasing the risk of phytophotodermatitis [24, 25, 28, 31, 33]. In the spring or summer months, people may spend more time outdoors and wear clothing with less skin coverage. Caucasians may have a greater risk to phytophotodermatitis than African Americans, possibly related to having less of the protective effect of pigmentation or other photoprotective mechanism in the epidermis [56].

There are also factors that can enhance photoreactivity. Higher intensity light, heat, hydration (humidity, swimming, bathing), infections, open wounds, contact time with a plant, and contact with specific plant parts, could all enhance absorption and degree of damage [4, 11–13, 40, 52].

In terms of creating a strategy to educate the public, the method of communication can play an important role. In the previously discussed study by Rzymski and colleagues, it is shown that the common sources of information, from the most to least, are internet, television, school, press, friends, radio, professional literature, flyers, and social campaigns [11].

Clinical Diseases Caused by Plant Exposure

The inflammatory reaction of phytophotodermatitis can begin minutes after exposure and peak at around 48 hours [4, 7, 11]. The lesions are described as well-demarcated erythematous, edematous, dusky plaques, which often develop vesicles or bullae [4]. The lesions are typically painful or burning, more than pruritic, which can be an important characteristic in differentiating the eruption from allergic contact dermatitis (e.g. Toxicodendron dermatitis) [3, 41, 57]. Subsequently, post-inflammatory hyperpigmentation can develop and last for months or even years, and sensitivity to ultraviolet light can persist [4, 11, 54]. Several recent cases documented hypopigmentation resulting from phytophotodermatitis [4, 41]. Seldom, isolated pigmentation can be the only presenting symptom as observed in two recent cases [21]. This is thought to be due to low- dose photosensitizer and/or UVA concentrations that do not elicit an observable inflammatory response [12, 21]. Alternatively, extreme cases can present, as did a rare case of full thickness burn and necrosis with secondary superinfection resulting in leg amputation [58].

The pattern of skin involvement may aid in the diagnosis. The lesions can occur in various patterns, including non-dermatomal, bizarre, or linear distribution but should relate to contact with plant photosensitizer [4]. Patients may develop a lip or hand reaction if there is oral or manual contact with a lime during the process of alcohol consumption [3]. In previously described cases, photosensitive substances have been inadvertently applied to children by unknowing parents after squeezing limes, resulting in digitate, loop-shaped, or irregular hyperpigmentation mimicking child abuse [65]. Strimmer dermatitis (weed-whacker dermatitis) results from the use of a high velocity powered gardening device and can present with widely scattered macules and papules on the anterior chest, arms, or legs, where plant debris contacted the skin [59]. Berlock (or Berloque) dermatitis results from plant photosensitizing- containing cologne or fragrance that is applied and classically results in streaks of pigmentation running down the neck with increase pigment toward the lower portion [60]. The appearance is that of a pendant or watch chain [60]. Modern day misting sprays may present in a more diffuse photodistributed pattern (Fig. 1a, b).

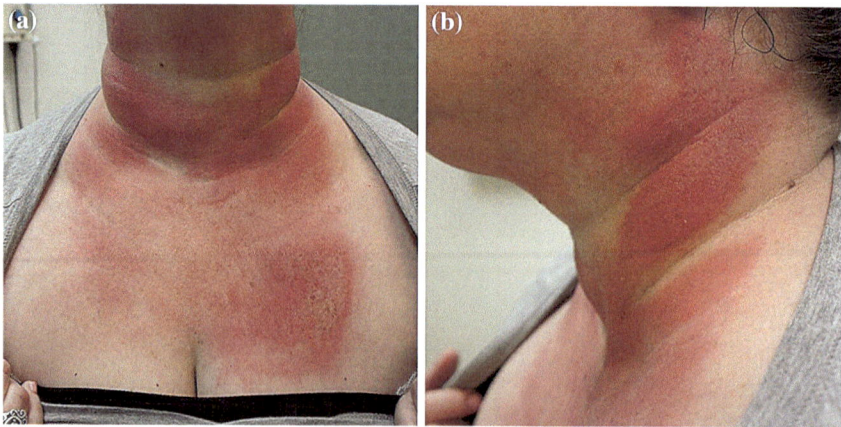

Fig. 1 **a** Berloque dermatitis characterized by erythematous patches in photodistributed pattern on a women's neck and chest (Photo credit courtesy of Harry Dao, MD, Baylor College of Medicine Department of Dermatology.). **b** Lateral view of same patient in (**a**) (Photo credit courtesy of Harry Dao, MD, Baylor College of Medicine Department of Dermatology.)

Diagnosis

The diagnosis of phytophotodermatitis is generally made on a clinical basis. The history is of utmost importance in identifying exposures to phototoxic plants and UVA radiation. Photopatch testing and biopsy can be performed to confirm the reaction and provide additional information [4, 7, 61]. Neither is necessary for diagnosis.

The differential diagnosis can be challenging as plants can also cause irritant contact dermatitis and allergic contact dermatitis [7]. Plants often contain other compounds that can cause these conditions to co-exist and some speculate that furocoumarins themselves may have a photoallergy effect [7, 61, 62]. Other diagnoses to consider are infectious (e.g., cellulitis, herpes simplex virus, tinea), vesiculobullous disorders, drug reactions, or photosensitivity disorders (e.g., polymorphous light eruption, solar urticaria, porphyrias, pellagra) [7, 63, 64]. An important differential diagnosis that must be considered is non-accidental injury to a child [63, 65].

Treatment

The treatment team is an important consideration and may include multiple disciplines including emergency medicine, dermatology, burn units and plastic surgery. The lesions can essentially be considered varying degrees of a chemical burn and would need to be continually assessed [3].

First steps in therapy are the removal and avoidance of any phototoxic agent and/or ultraviolet radiation. The area should be washed with soap and water as soon as exposure is recognized. As pain is a common symptom, some patients may need analgesic treatment with nonsteroidal anti-inflammatory drugs or opioids [4, 13]. If inflammation is evident with erythema or edema, topical steroids can help control symptoms [3, 4, 13]. Sunscreens are recommended to protect against further damage and for the increased sensitivity of the skin after toxic insult [3]. Activities that promote moisture exposure (e.g. swimming) can aggravate lesions and should be avoided [4, 13].

When blistering has occurred, additional management is needed. Debridement is generally considered for ruptured blisters while intact blister debridement is controversial [66]. Risk and benefit analysis for consideration of debridement include need for wound depth assessment, infection risk, moisture balance, mechanical pressure, healing, lesion location, impact on function, application of dressings and medications, patient comfort and experience of the clinician [66]. Small blisters can be drained with a sterile needle [13]. With superficial partial-thickness involvement, large bullae can be unroofed and cleansed (e.g. chlorhexidine) and provided with application of topical antibiotic prophylaxis (e.g. silver sulfadiazine) and wound dressings [13]. The wound dressing can reduce pain, aid re-epithelization and healing and protect from infection and UV radiation [13]. Dressings that have been used include simple and perforated, non-adherent dressings, petrolatum-impregnated gauze, potassium permanganate-impregnated dressings, silver-containing dressings (e.g. Acticoat), paraffin dressings (e.g., Tulle gras, Bactigras), and synthetic resorbable skin substitute (e.g. Suprathel) [4, 13, 67–69]. If edema is present, pressure bandages over wound dressings can be utilized. Moisturizing cream or ointment may be beneficial after wound dressing.

Severe cases would prompt hospital admission, intravenous fluid replacement, systemic steroids, and referral to a burn unit [13]. General sedation and analgesia may be needed in the burn unit to facilitate inspection of the wounds [13]. Full-thickness involvement may necessitate skin grafting and possible amputation if necessary [58, 70]. Continual monitoring for secondary infections is essential and may warrant the need for systemic antibiotics [3].

Hyperpigmentation has been treated with topical steroids, hydroquinone, and tretinoin to help reduce undesirable discoloration [4, 18, 71]. Continued sun avoidance and protection is crucial and cosmetic camouflage can be utilized [4].

Preventative Measures

Recognition of phytophotodermatitis and implicated plants is an important method to prevent disease. The prevention of phytophotodermatitis is accomplished by avoiding exposures to the plant toxins. Market trends ("natural" products) in the cosmetic, aromatherapy, and food industries should receive special attention to identify potentially photosensitizing ingredients used in new products [34]. Lawn management (e.g. mowing, herbicides) may prevent growth and spread of implicated plants [11]. With outside activities, such as lawn care or playtime for children, proper protective clothing is important (e.g., full-length shirts and pants, gloves, sunglasses, hats) [11]. If there has been contact with known photosensitizing plants, washing the skin with soap and water is crucial to remove the offending agent before activation [4]. Even if photosensitizing agents have not been removed, avoiding sunlight and sun protection can prevent activation of photosensitizers [4]. Patients should avoid occlusion with creams and/or ointments before consulting a physician, as these may enhance the phototoxic effect [58].

Declaration of Interest The authors have no conflict of interest to declare.

Informed Consent Obtained written consent.

References

1. Klaber R. Phyto-photo-dermatitis. Br J Dermatol. 1942;54(7):193–211. https://doi.org/10.1111/j.1365-2133.1942.tb10682.x.
2. Pathak MA, Fitzpatrick TB. The evolution of photochemotherapy with psoralens and UVA (PUVA): 2000 BC to 1992 AD. J Photochem Photobiol, B. 1992;14(1–2):3–22. ,

3. Bowers AG. Phytophotodermatitis. Am J Contact Dermat. 1999;10(2):89–93. https://doi. org/10.1016/S1046-199X(99)90006-4.

4. Baker BG, Bedford J, Kanitkar S. Keeping pace with the media; Giant Hogweed burns—a case series and comprehensive review. Burns J Int Soc Burn Inj. 2017;43(5):933–8. https:// doi.org/10.1016/j.burns.2016.10.018.

5. Giant hogweed 'UK's most dangerous plant', say rivers trust. BBC News. https://www.bbc. com/news/uk-england-manchester-33509053. Accessed 2 Feb 2019.

6. Chaudhary SK, Ceska O, Warrington PJ, Ashwood-Smith MJ. Increased furocoumarin content of celery during storage. J Agric Food Chem. 1985;33(6):1153–7. https://doi. org/10.1021/jf00066a032.

7. Son JH, Jin H, You HS, Shim WH, Kim JM, Kim GW, et al. Five cases of phytophotoder-matitis caused by fig leaves and relevant literature review. Ann Dermatol. 2017;29(1):86–90. https://doi.org/10.5021/ad.2017.29.1.86.

8. Zangerl AR, Berenbaum MR. Increase in toxicity of an invasive weed after reassociation with its coevolved herbivore. Proc Natl Acad Sci USA. 2005;102(43):15529–32. https://doi. org/10.1073/pnas.0507805102.

9. Seligman PJ, Mathias CG, O'Malley MA, Beier RC, Fehrs LJ, Serrill WS, et al. Phytophotodermatitis from celery among grocery store workers. Arch Dermatol. 1987;123(11):1478–82.

10. Fu PP, Xia Q, Zhao Y, Wang S, Yu H, Chiang HM. Phototoxicity of herbal plants and herbal products. J Environ Sci Health, Part C Environ Carcinog Ecotoxicol Rev. 2013;31(3):213–55. https://doi.org/10.1080/10590501.2013.824206.

11. Rzymski P, Klimaszyk P, Poniedzialek B. Invasive giant hogweeds in Poland: Risk of burns among forestry workers and plant distribution. Burns. 2015;41(8):1816–22. https://doi. org/10.1016/j.burns.2015.06.007.

12. Knudsen EA, Kroon S. In vitro and in vivo phototoxicity of furocoumarin-containing plants. Clin Exp Dermatol. 1988;13(2):92–6.

13. Pfurtscheller K, Trop M. Phototoxic plant burns: report of a case and review of topical wound treatment in children. Pediatr Dermatol. 2014;31(6):e156–9. https://doi.org/10.1111/ pde.12396.

14. Crosby DG. The poisoned weed: plants toxic to skin. Oxford: Oxford University Press; 2004.

15. Kabuce N, Priede N. NOBANIS—Invasive alien species fact sheet—Heracleum sos-nowskyi. In: Online database of the European network on invasive alien species. NOBANIS; 2010. www.nobanis.org. Accessed 2 Feb 2019.

16. An I, Ozturk M. Phytodermatitis in east and southeast of Turkey: a prospective study. Cutan Ocul Toxicol. 2018:1–19. https://doi.org/10.1080/15569527.2018.1561711.

17. Dufayet L, Langrand J. Phytophotodermatitis related to Peucedanum paniculatum Loisel, a case report. Contact Dermat. 2018. https://doi.org/10.1111/cod.13185.

18. Bosanac SS, Clark AK, Sivamani RK. Phytophotodermatitis related to carrot extract-con-taining sunscreen. Derm Online J. 2018;24(1).

19. Zhang RZ, Zhu WY. Phytophotodermatitis due to wild carrot decoction. Indian J Dermtol, Venereol Leprol. 2011;77(6):731. https://doi.org/10.4103/0378-6323.86511.

20. Izumi AK, Dawson KL. Zabon phytophotodermatitis: first case reports due to Citrus max-ima. J Am Acad Dermatol. 2002;46(5 Suppl):S146–7.

21. Choi JY, Hwang S, Lee SH, Oh SH. Asymptomatic hyperpigmentation without preced-ing inflammation as a clinical feature of citrus fruits-induced phytophotodermatitis. Ann Dermatol. 2018;30(1):75–8. https://doi.org/10.5021/ad.2018.30.1.75.

22. Fitzpatrick JK, Kohlwes J. Lime-induced phytophotodermatitis. J Gen Intern Med. 2018;33(6):975. https://doi.org/10.1007/s11606-018-4315-z.

23. Friedman BT, Harper R, Glucksberg A, Strote J. In the limelight. J Emerg Med. 2016;50(3):504–5. https://doi.org/10.1016/j.jemermed.2015.11.014.

24. Harshman J, Quan Y, Hsiang D. Phytophotodermatitis: rash with many faces. Can Fam Physician Med Fam Can. 2017;63(12):938–40.

25. Kristiansen B, Penninga L, Diernaes JEF. Challenging cause of bullous eruption of the hands in the Arctic. BMJ Case Rep. 2018;2018. https://doi.org/10.1136/bcr-2018-225981.

26. Marcos LA, Kahler R. Phytophotodermatitis. Int J Infect Dis: IJID: Off Publ Int Soc Infect Dis. 2015;38:7–8. https://doi.org/10.1016/j.ijid.2015.07.004.

27. Matthews MR, VanderVelde JC, Caruso DM, Foster KN. Lemons in the arizona sunshine: the effects of furocoumarins leading to phytophotodermatitis and burn-like injuries. Wounds: Compend Clin Res Pract. 2017;29(12):E118–e24.

28. Mioduszewski M, Beecker J. Phytophotodermatitis from making sangria: a phototoxic reaction to lime and lemon juice. CMAJ. 2015;187(10):756. https://doi.org/10.1503/cmaj.140942.

29. Raam R, DeClerck B, Jhun P, Herbert M. Phytophotodermatitis: the other "lime" disease. Ann Emerg Med. 2016;67(4):554–6. https://doi.org/10.1016/j.annemergmed.2016.02.023.

30. Safran T, Kanevsky J, Ferland-Caron G, Mereniuk A, Perreault I, Lee J. Blistering phytophotodermatitis of the hands after contact with lime juice. Contact Dermat. 2017;77(1):53–4. https://doi.org/10.1111/cod.12728.

31. Schmitt AR, Bellamkonda VR. Man With Right Hand Bullae. Ann Emerg Med. 2016;67(4):553, 6. https://doi.org/10.1016/j.annemergmed.2015.07.502.

32. Snaidr VA, Lowe PM. Phytophotodermatitis from lime juice. Med J Aust. 2017;207(8):328.

33. Torres-Navarro I, Condino-Brito E, Botella-Estrada R. "Mojito's" phytophotodermatitis, the other "lime" disease. Med Clin. 2018;151(1):44. https://doi.org/10.1016/j.medcli.2017.08.008.

34. Binder S, Hanakova A, Tomankova K, Pizova K, Bajgar R, Manisova B, et al. Adverse phototoxic effect of essential plant oils on NIH 3T3 cell line after UV light exposure. Cent Eur J Public Health. 2016;24(3):234–40. https://doi.org/10.21101/cejph.a4354.

35. Machado M, Vidal RL, Cardoso P, Coelho S. Phytophotodermatitis: a diagnosis to consider. BMJ case reports. 2015;2015. https://doi.org/10.1136/bcr-2015-213388.

36. Cordoba S, Gonzalez M, Martinez-Moran C, Borbujo JM. Bullous phytophotodermatitis caused by an esoteric remedy. Actas Dermo-Sifiliograficas. 2017;108(1):79–81. https://doi.org/10.1016/j.ad.2016.07.019.

37. Gawkrodger DJ, Savin JA. Phytophotodermatitis due to common rue (*Ruta graveolens*). Contact Dermat. 1983;9(3):224.

38. Booth B, Furzeland J. An unusual rash for Royal: a case series. J R Nav Med Serv. 2016;102(1):19–21.

39. Mateus JE, Silva CD, Ferreira M, Porto J. Phytophotodermatitis: still a poorly recognised diagnosis. BMJ Case Rep. 2018;2018:bcr-2018-227859. https://doi.org/10.1136/bcr-2018-227859.

40. Zaynoun ST, Aftimos BG, Abi Ali L, Tenekjian KK, Khalidi U, Kurban AK. Ficus carica; isolation and quantification of the photoactive components. Contact Dermat. 1984;11(1):21–5.

41. Rademaker M, Derraik JG. Phytophotodermatitis caused by Ficus pumila. Contact Dermat. 2012;67(1):53–6. https://doi.org/10.1111/j.1600-0536.2012.02026.x.

42. Beattie PE, Dawe RS, Traynor NJ, Woods JA, Ferguson J, Ibbotson SH. Can St John's wort (hypericin) ingestion enhance the erythemal response during high-dose ultraviolet al therapy? Br J Dermato. 2005;153(6):1187–91. https://doi.org/10.1111/j.1365-2133.2005.06946.x.

43. Hohmann N, Maus A, Carls A, Haefeli WE, Mikus G. St. John's wort treatment in women bears risks beyond pharmacokinetic drug interactions. Arch Toxicol. 2016;90(4):1013–5. https://doi.org/10.1007/s00204-015-1532-7.

44. Napoli E, Siracusa L, Ruberto G, Carrubba A, Lazzara S, Speciale A, et al. Phytochemical profiles, phototoxic and antioxidant properties of eleven Hypericum species—a comparative study. Phytochemistry. 2018;152:162–73. https://doi.org/10.1016/j.phytochem.2018.05.003.

45. Alam F, Khan GN, Asad M. Psoralea corylifolia L: ethnobotanical, biological, and chemical aspects: a review. Phytother Res PTR. 2018;32(4):597–615. https://doi.org/10.1002/ptr.6006.

46. Maurice PD, Cream JJ. The dangers of herbalism. BMJ (Clinical research ed). 1989;299(6709):1204-.

47. Ozkol HU, Akdeniz N, Ozkol H, Bilgili SG, Calka O. Development of phytophotodermatitis in two cases related to Plantago lanceolata. Cutan Ocul Toxicol. 2012;31(1):58–60. https://doi.org/10.3109/15569527.2011.584232.

48. Ozkol HU, Calka O, Akdeniz N, Pinar SM. Phytodermatitis in eastern Turkey: a retrospective, observational study. Dermat Contact Atopic Occup Drug. 2014;25(3):140–6. https://doi.org/10.1097/der.0000000000000033.

49. Pyšek P, Chytry M, Pergl J, Sádlo J, Wild J. Plant invasions in the Czech Republic: current state, introduction dynamics, invasive species and invaded habitats. 2012.

50. Zavaleta E. The economic value of controlling an invasive shrub. SPIE; 2000.

51. Lenkovic M, Cabrijan L, Gruber F, Saftic M, Stanic Zgombic Z, Stasic A, et al. Phytophotodermatitis in Rijeka region, Croatia. CollIum Antropol. 2008;32(Suppl 2):203–5.

52. Zobel AM, Brown SA. Seasonal changes of furanocoumarin concentrations in leaves of *Heracleum lanatum*. J Chem Ecol. 1990;16(5):1623–34. https://doi.org/10.1007/bf01014095.

53. Zhang R, Zhu W. Phytophotodermatitis due to chinese herbal medicine decoction. Indian J Dermato. 2011;56(3):329–31. https://doi.org/10.4103/0019-5154.82498.

54. Van Wyk B-E, Wink M. Phytomedicines, herbal drugs, and poisons. Chicago: University of Chicago Press; 2014.

55. Dobson J, Ondhia C, Skellett AM, Coelho R. Image gallery: phototoxic rash from celery diet. Br J Dermato. 2016;175(5):e133. https://doi.org/10.1111/bjd.14980.

56. Nakamura M, Henderson M, Jacobsen G, Lim HW. Comparison of photodermatoses in African-Americans and Caucasians: a follow-up study. Photodermatol Photoimmunol Photomed. 2014;30(5):231–6. https://doi.org/10.1111/phpp.12079.

57. Kruse LL. Differential diagnosis of linear eruptions in children. Pediatr Ann. 2015;44(8):e194–8. https://doi.org/10.3928/00904481-20150812-08.

58. Klimaszyk P, Klimaszyk D, Piotrowiak M, Popiolek A. Unusual complications after occupational exposure to giant hogweed (Heracleum mantegazzianum): a case report. Int J Occup Med Environ Health. 2014;27(1):141–4. https://doi.org/10.2478/s13382-014-0238-z.

59. Reynolds NJ, Burton JL, Bradfield JWB, Matthews CNA. Weed wacker dermatitis. Arch Dermatol. 1991;127(9):1419–20. https://doi.org/10.1001/archderm.1991.01680080159028.

60. Lane JE, Strauss MJ. Toilet water dermatitis: with especial reference to berlock dermatitis. J Am Med Assoc. 1930;95(10):717–9. https://doi.org/10.1001/jama.1930.02720100015005.

61. Bonamonte D, Foti C, Lionetti N, Rigano L, Angelini G. Photoallergic contact dermatitis to 8-methoxypsoralen in Ficus carica. Contact Dermat. 2010;62(6):343–8. https://doi.org/10.1111/j.1600-0536.2010.01713.x.

62. Jakubska-Busse A, Michał Ś, Kobyłka M. Identification of bioactive components of essential oils in Heracleum sosnowskyi and Heracleum mantegazzianum (Apiaceae). 2013.

63. Carlsen K, Weismann K. Phytophotodermatitis in 19 children admitted to hospital and their differential diagnoses: Child abuse and herpes simplex virus infection. J Am Acad Dermatol. 2007;57(5 Suppl):S88–91. https://doi.org/10.1016/j.jaad.2006.08.034.

64. Gould JW, Mercurio MG, Elmets CA. Cutaneous photosensitivity diseases induced by exogenous agents. J Am Acad Dermatol. 1995;33(4):551–73; quiz 74-6.

65. Coffman K, Boyce WT, Hansen RC. Phytophotodermatitis simulating child abuse. Am J Dis Child. 1985;139(3):239–40. https://doi.org/10.1001/archpedi.1985.02140050033015.

66. Sargent RL. Management of blisters in the partial-thickness burn: an integrative research review. J Burn Care Res Off Publ Am Burn Assoc. 2006;27(1):66–81. https://doi.org/10.1097/01.bcr.0000191961.95907.b1.

67. Probert SM, Lacey J, Gautam S. Giant Hogweed burns. Arch Dis Child. 2013;98(7):544. https://doi.org/10.1136/archdischild-2012-303229.
68. Mill J, Wallis B, Cuttle L, Mott J, Oakley A, Kimble R. Phytophotodermatitis: case reports of children presenting with blistering after preparing lime juice. Burns J Int Soc Burn Inj. 2008;34(5):731–3. https://doi.org/10.1016/j.burns.2007.11.010.
69. Mandalia MR, Chalmers R, Schreuder FB. Contact with fig tree sap: an unusual cause of burn injury. Burns J Int Soc Burn Inj. 2008;34(5):719–21. https://doi.org/10.1016/j.burns.2007.03.026.
70. Chan JC, Sullivan PJ, O'Sullivan MJ, Eadie PA. Full thickness burn caused by exposure to giant hogweed: delayed presentation, histological features and surgical management. J Plast Reconstr Aesthetic Surg JPRAS. 2011;64(1):128–30. https://doi.org/10.1016/j.bjps.2010.03.030.
71. Phytophototoxin Poisoning Treatment & Management. https://emedicine.medscape.com/article/817226-treatment. Accessed 2 Oct 2019.
72. Dean FM. Naturally Occurring Coumarins. In: Zechmeister L, editor. Fortschritte der Chemie Organischer Naturstoffe (Progress in the Chemistry of Organic Natural Products/Progrès Dans La Chimie Des Substances Organiques Naturelles). Vienna: Springer Vienna; 1952. p. 225–91.
73. Murray RDH. Naturally occurring plant coumarins. In: Herz W, Grisebach H, Kirby GW, editors. Fortschritte der Chemie Organischer Naturstoffe (Progress in the chemistry of organic natural products). Vienna: Springer Vienna; 1978. p. 199–429.
74. Murray RDH. Naturally occurring plant coumarins. In: Herz W, Kirby GW, Steglich W, Tamm C, editors. Fortschritte der Chemie organischer Naturstoffe (Progress in the chemistry of organic natural products). Vienna: Springer Vienna; 1991. p. 83–316.
75. Murray RDH. Naturally occurring plant coumarins. Fortschritte der Chemie organischer Naturstoffe (Progress in the chemistry of organic natural products). Vienna: Springer Vienna; 1997. p. 1–119.
76. Murray RDH. The naturally occurring coumarins. In: Herz W, Falk H, Kirby GW, Moore RE, editors. Fortschritte der Chemie organischer Naturstoffe (Progress in the chemistry of organic natural products). Vienna: Springer Vienna; 2002. p. 1–619.
77. Sarker SD, Nahar L. Progress in the chemistry of naturally occurring coumarins. In: Kinghorn AD, Falk H, Gibbons S, Kobayashi JI, editors. Progress in the chemistry of organic natural products 106. Cham: Springer International Publishing; 2017. p. 241–304.

Allergic Contact Dermatitis Due to Plants

Gillian Weston and Amy Y-Y Chen

Introduction and Features of Allergic Contact Dermatitis

Allergic contact dermatitis (ACD) is one of the most common entities encountered not only by dermatologists but also by other healthcare providers. However, the true incidence of ACD is difficult to estimate [13]. ACD is a type IV, delayed hypersensitivity reaction that occurs as a result of contact with a culprit allergen. When the allergen contacts the skin of a sensitized individual, antigen-specific T-helper cells are activated, leading to a downstream inflammatory response [13].

Plants can cause ACD with potential allergens found in everyday environments including the home, garden, recreational and occupational settings [41]. Patients presenting with ACD due to plants often present with well-demarcated pruritic, erythematous, edematous vesicular or scaly papules and plaques on exposed skin. A linear configuration of lesions is common, correlating with a brush against a culprit plant. In the following sections, the most important and frequently-encountered plants which induce ACD are discussed.

Anacardiaceae Family

The most well-known plant that causes ACD is the toxicodendron species of the anacardiaceae family which includes poison ivy, poison oak and poison sumac. This species was formerly thought to be part of the *rhus* genus, and the resultant

G. Weston (✉)
263 Farmington Ave, Farmington, CT 06030-6231, USA
e-mail: gweston@uchc.edu

A.Y-Y. Chen
Central Connecticut Dermatology, 1 Willowbrook Rd, Suite #2, Cromwell, CT 06416, USA
e-mail: ayyen@alum.mit.edu

© Springer Nature Switzerland AG 2020
J. Trevino and A.Y-Y. Chen (eds.), *Dermatological Manual of Outdoor Hazards*,
https://doi.org/10.1007/978-3-030-37782-3_5

dermatitis was called "rhus dermatitis". However, toxicodendron species are now thought to represent their own genus. Millions of North Americans are affected every year as a result of contact with these species. In fact, contact dermatitis is a major cause of occupational dermatitis with the highest rate occurring in those in the agriculture, forestry and firefighting industries [19, 32]. It is estimated that as much as 75% of the United States adult population is sensitized to plants in the anacardiaceae family with only 10% considered tolerant to the responsible allergen [19]. Various other, but less commonly known, allergenic species in this family include the cashew nut tree, mango tree, Brazilian pepper tree, Japanese lacquer tree and Indian marking tree nut. Descriptions and epidemiology of each species can be found below, followed by discussion of the allergenic compounds produced by this family of plants.

Toxicodendron species

Toxicodendron radicans, otherwise known as northern poison ivy or eastern poison ivy, is a perennial native to the continental United States (US) and Canada, east of the Rocky Mountains [49]. Each leaf contains three leaflets, alternating along the main vein as depicted in Fig. 1. The central leaflet has a stem that is longer than the stems of the two lateral leaflets. Older plants tend to have a hairy stem and may bear green fruit (Fig. 2) that turns off-white as it ages [17].

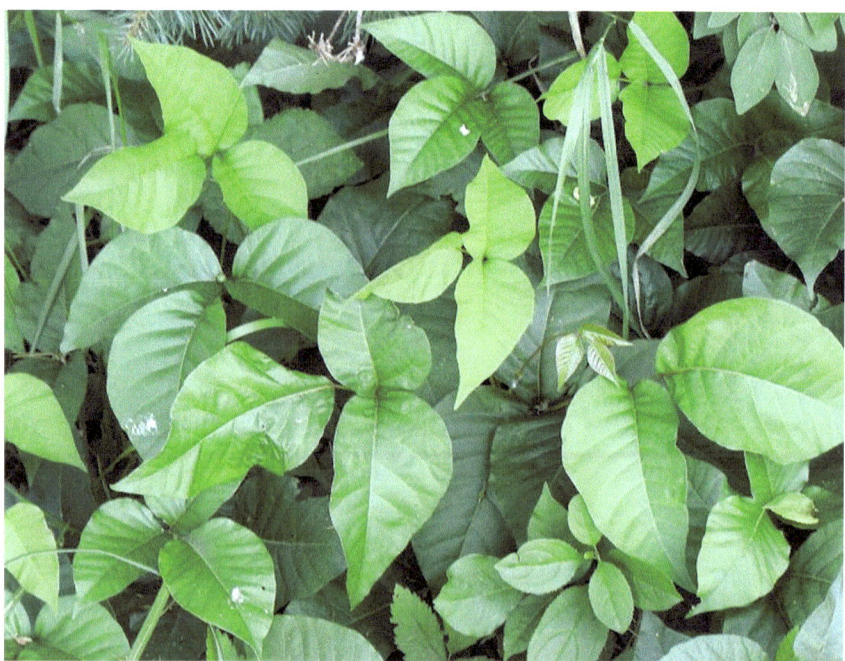

Fig. 1 *Toxicodendron radicans.* Photo courtesy of: Esculapio (https://commons.wikimedia.org/wiki/File:Toxicodendron_radicans.jpg), "Toxicodendron radicans", marked as public domain, more details on Wikimedia Commons: https://commons.wikimedia.org/wiki/Template:PD-user

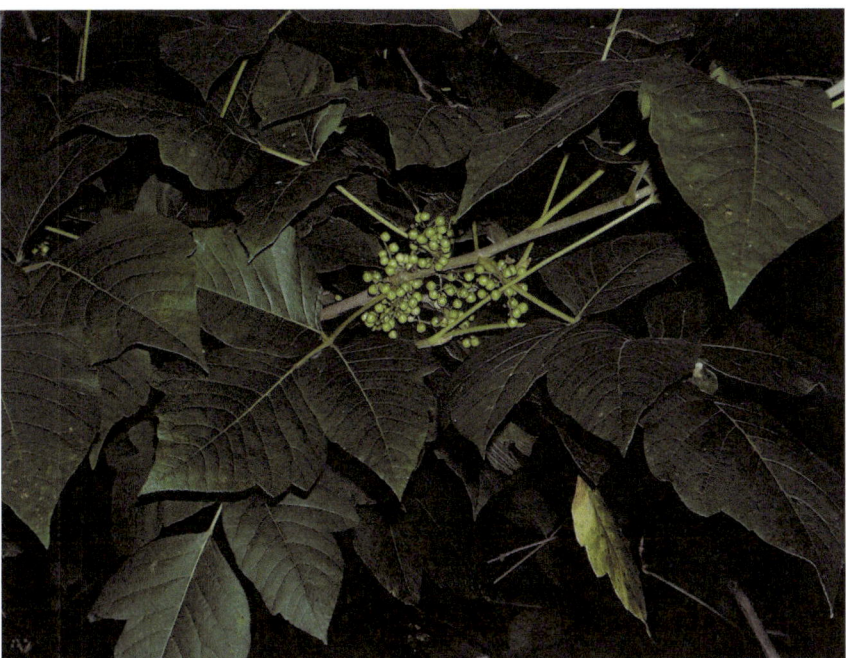

Fig. 2 *Toxicodendron radicans bearing green fruit.* Photo courtesy of: Jvlietstra (https://commons.wikimedia.org/wiki/File:Poison_Ivy_Berries.JPG), "Poison Ivy Berries", marked as public domain, more details on Wikimedia Commons: https://commons.wikimedia.org/wiki/Template:PD-user

Toxicodendron rydbergii, commonly referred to as western poison ivy, is also a perennial that is native in Canada and most of the continental US with the exception of the southeastern US and California [49]. Leaves are similar to those of *T. radicans*.

Toxicodendron toxicarium, referred to as eastern poison oak, is a woody perennial native to the southeastern US [49]. It typically has three leaflets similar to those of the *T. radicans* species [35].

Toxicodendron diversilobum, known as western poison oak or pacific poison oak, is a perennial shrub or vine native to the west coast of the continental US and Canada [49]. Leaves may have 3 or 5 leaflets which are irregularly lobed, similar in appearance to an oak leaf. The plant produces green or off-white flowers and white fruits [4].

Toxicodendron venix, colloquially known as poison sumac (Fig. 3), is a perennial shrub that is native to the eastern part of North America, primarily found in shaded, swampy areas [49]. The plant bears white or green hanging fruits and has leaves, each with 7–13 leaflets.

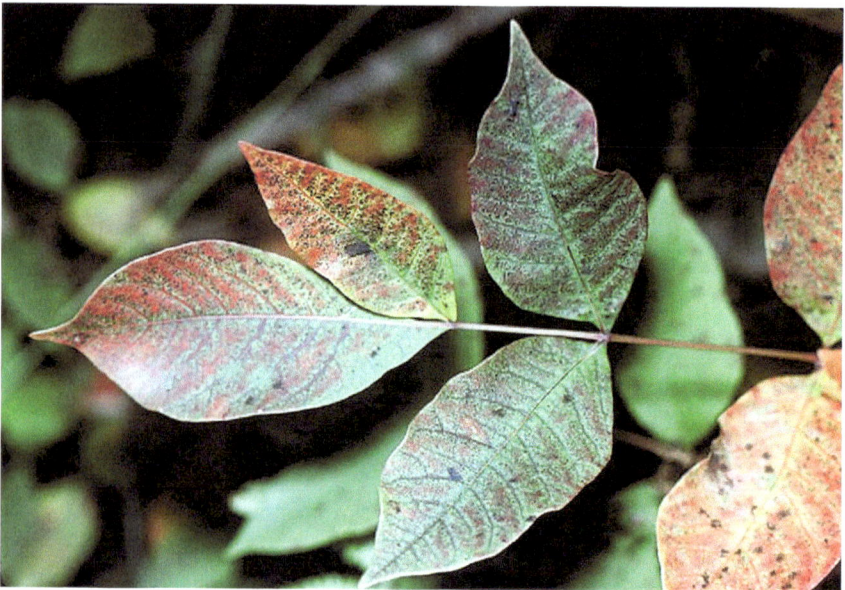

Fig. 3 *Toxicodendron vernix*. Photo courtesy of: (https://commons.wikimedia.org/wiki/File:-Toxicodendron_vernix.jpg), "Toxicodendron vernix", marked as public domain, more details on Wikimedia Commons: https://commons.wikimedia.org/wiki/Template:PD-US

Toxicodendron vernicifluum, known as the Chinese lacquer tree or the Japanese lacquer tree, is native to parts of China, Japan and Korea. While it is not native to North America, it may be used in domestic landscaping [39].

Other species

Schinus terebinthifolius, known as the Brazilian peppertree, Florida holly or the Christmas berry tree, is perennial shrub or tree native to the southern continental US, Hawaii, Puerto Rico and the US Virgin Islands [48]. Interestingly, it is prohibited in Florida as it produces thick stems that potentially shade and displace other rare native plant species [50]. It yields a dark green leaves with 3–11 leaflets, which when crushed produce an aroma similar to that of pepper or turpentine. It bears white flowers with 5 petals and red berries [50].

The mango tree, *Mangifera indica*, is a perennial tree native to the state of Florida, among other warmer climates outside the US. Mango trees can be easily identified as they bear the characteristic irregularly egg-shaped fruit with green, yellow or red skin overlying a yellow-orange sweet flesh [47]. The trees are tall, up to 30 meters in height, and are narrow. They bear leathery, oblong, alternating leaves [47].

Anacardium occidentale, or the cashew nut tree, which originated in Brazil, is native to Puerto Rico and the US Virgin Islands [46]. Trees have a domed canopy with sparse, leathery, dark green leaves limited to the distal branches. It produces a kidney shaped nut inside a brown shell which grows off of a fleshy yellow pear shaped accessory fruit, colloquially known as the cashew apple.

The Indian marking nut tree, *Semecarpus anacardium*, is native to warmer parts of India where it is commonly used in Ayruvedic medicine. These trees can reach 25 meters in height with trunks bearing grey flaking bark and oblong leaves. It also bears green or white fruit similar to other members of the *anacardiaceae* family [43].

The gluta rengas tree, also a member of the anacardiaceae family, is native to Southeast Asia.. It produces an edible seed and its wood is used in building furniture and other wooden items.

Anacardiaceae- induced allergic contact dermatitis

Urushiol is the allergen present in plants of the anacardiaceae family responsible for ACD. It is present in the oleoresin of the plants and can be on and within the leaves, vines, stems and roots [51]. Urushiol is a mixture of pentadecylcatechols [19]. Although the urushiol differs slightly among plants in the anacardiaceae family, they are structurally similar enough that they cross-react. An individual who is sensitive to one plant is sensitive to all plants within the family [19]. Urushiol is released when any part of the plant is damaged and when released, it dries quickly. However, it remains allergenic in its dry state [16]. When exposed to air, urushiol is oxidized and turns from colorless or slightly yellow to black, causing "black spot poison ivy" when oxidized on the skin [12]. Herbal products derived from the anacardiaceae family can cause systemic contact dermatitis if ingested by individuals sensitized to urushiol [30].

Diagnosis

History, including thorough exposure history and physical examination are typically sufficient to make a diagnosis of ACD. Further testing is usually not necessarily. However, plant oleoresin can be diluted with acetone and used in patch testing if needed.

Cross Reactions

Various plants of alternative families may cross react in those who are sensitive to urushiol.. These include African poison ivy (*Smodingium argutum*) and the ginkgo tree (*Ginkgo biloba* of the gingoaceae family) [19].

Compositae Family

The compositae, or asteraceae family is another group of plants that are common causes of ACD. It is one of the largest plant families with species distributed all over the world. Members of this family have flowering heads composed of many florets, or small flowers. Florets are surrounded by leaf-like structures called bracts [45]. The stems bear leaves of various arrangements.

The compositae family is found in a variety of settings. Common garden plants in this family include chrysanthemums, dahlias, marigolds, feverfew chamomile, daisies, gerbera, zinnias, burdock, butterbur, calendula, cat's ear, cudweed, hawksbeard and arnica. Noxious weeds such as dandelions, ragweed and thistles are also members of this family. Furthermore, several food crops also belong to the compositae family, including artichokes, lettuce, endive, chicory, escarole and salsify. Edible seeds from compositae family members safflower and sunflower are used to make cooking oils. Wormwood, another member, is used in making absinthe liqueur [45].

Compositae- induced allergic contact dermatitis

In addition to the typical localized ACD at sites of contact, plants in the compositae family are the leading cause of airborne ACD which often presents with eyelid, neck or facial dermatitis. Involvement of non-sun exposed skin including the post-auricular neck and submental neck can help differentiate airborne ACD from photodermatitis. Sensitized patients who ingest components of a plant from this family may develop oral swelling or a systemic contact dermatitis.

The allergens in the compositae family are sesquiterpene lactones (SQL). SQLs are a group of metabolites found in plants of the compositae family and other plants including those in the cactaceae, solanaceae, araceae and eurphorbiaceae families. SQLs are colorless, lipophilic lactones. They generally have a cyclic 15 carbon backbone and are synthesized and modified by various enzymes resulting in an extensive array of different SQLs [11].

Diagnosis

Although thorough exposure history is sufficient to diagnose ACD due to SQL-containing plants, patch testing is available to aid in diagnosis. Due to the sheer number of different SQLs, no single ideal patch testing material exists. A mix of 3 of the main 6 structural components of SQLs are part of one mix developed by Benezra and Epstein, which has been able to identify 60% of sensitized individuals [37]. Compositae mix is a mixture of arnica, yarrow, tansy, chamomile and feverfew; it may detect more cases but can also cause sensitization in previously unsensitized individuals or cause an irritant contact dermatitis (ICD) [52].

Cross Reactions

Patients who are sensitized to one plant within the compositae family are likely to cross- react to other plants in the family. Although the specific culprit SQL may be different, overall SQLs are similar enough to activate sensitized T cells. Permethrin is the most important cross-reactor to be aware of as it is often prescribed for scabies or pediculosis infestation. Topical permethrin should therefore be avoided in patients with known sensitization to plants of the compositae family. Other species that produce SQLs include liverworts of the *Frullania species* in the *Jubulaceae family*, [41], *Para*-phenylenediamine (PPD), although structurally not similar to SQLs, has been reported to cross react in some SQL–sensitized individuals [36].

Liliaceae Family

The liliaceae family is a family of flowering plants including herbs and shrubs, the most well-known of which are the lilies (*lilium species*) and tulips (*tulipa species*). Other members include asparagus and hyacinth. Members of the family typically have flowers with six-segments and leaves clustered at the base of the plant [7].

Lilliaceae- induced allergic contact dermatitis

Contact dermatitis due to plants of liliaceae family typically presents as hand dermatitis, favoring the fingertips of the first and second fingers on the dominant hand. So called "tulip fingers" is a combined ACD and irritant contct dermatitis (ICD) due to repeated exposure to tulips; it presents with painful, eroded or fissured erythematous papules and plaques affecting the fingertips and periunugal skin. Florists and those involved in the growing and distribution of tulip bulbs are at increased risk [41].

Glucosides within plants of the liliaceae family include tuliposides A and B which are weakly allergenic. However, when hydrolyzed to tulipalin A and B, they become highly sensitizing. Tuliposide A and tulipalin A, are the most clinically significant sensitizers and are found in higher concentrations in the flowers, leaves and stems, compared to the bulbs [41].

Diagnosis

Thorough occupational and exposure history as well as clinical exam is sufficient to make a diagnosis of ACD to tulips. No commercially available allergen exists for patch testing [21, 24].

Cross Reactions

Due to similarity in allergens, plants of the alstromeriaceae family, discussed below, are common cross-reactors with the liliaceae family.

Alstromeriaceae Family

The alstromeriaceae family consists mainly of two species: *Alstromeria aurea* (Fig. 4), an orange flower, and *Alstromeria ligtu* colloquially known as the Peruvian lily. Peruvian lilies have petals mottled with various shades of lilac or pink. They are grown as ornamental plants in many parts of the world.

Alstromeriaceae- induced allergic contact dermatitis

ACD due to Alstromeriaceae is similar to ACD due to plants in the liliaceae family. Florists are at high risk and often present with eczematous or vesicular eruption affecting the fingertips of the first and second finger of the dominant hand. If leaves are stripped manually, an eczematous or vesicular eruption on the palms may occur. The non-dominant hand can also be involved [41].

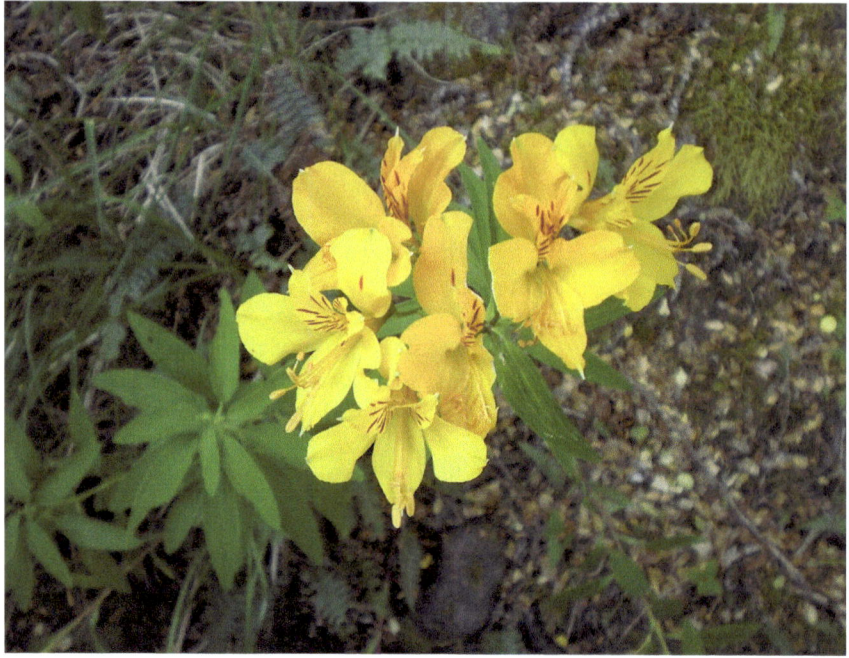

Fig. 4 *Alstromeria aurea*. Photo courtesy of: Claudio Elias (https://commons.wikimedia.org/wiki/File:Amancay001.JPG), "Amancay001", marked as public domain, more details on Wikimedia Commons: https://commons.wikimedia.org/wiki/Template:PD-self

The liliaceae and alstromeriaceae families share common allergens: α-methylene-γ-butyrolactones or tuliposides/tulipalin A [41]. They are found within the petals, leaves, stems and bulbs of the plant.

Diagnosis

As with ACD from other plants, history and physical is often sufficient for diagnosis. There is no commercially available allergen for patch testing.

Cross reactions

Due to the shared allergen, liliaceae species commonly cross–react in those sensitized to alstromeria species.

Proteaceae Family

The proteaceae family consists of *Grevillea species* including *Grevillea* commonly known as the southern silky oak, silk oak or silver oak and Grevillea Robyn Gordon which is a naturally occurring hybrid of two Grevillea species: *Grevillea banskii* and *Grevillea bipinnatifida*. These plants grow as low shrubs to tall forest trees and are native to the eastern coast of Australia as well as Hawaii and southern Florida. The silk oak tree is a tall, rugged evergreen with orange-yellow flowers which grows naturally in the forests. It is also planted ornamentally in warmer climates [44]. The Grevillea Robyn Gordon is a blooming shrub with large red-orange flowers and is the leading cause of plant-induced ACD in Australia [41].

Proteaceae- induced allergic contact dermatitis

Patients with ACD due to contact with proteaceae family present with eczematous, edematous and/or vesicular papules and plaques often in a linear configuration on exposed skin. Contact with the tree itself, and especially, its flowers or sawdust results in the characteristic eruption [40]. Sensitized individuals may also react when coming into contact with objects made of wood derived from other trees in this family [41].

Sensitizing agents are resorcinol derivatives and vary among specific species. A major component of some resorcinols is grevillol which is a phenolic compound with a long side chain that bears similarity to urushiol [22].

Diagnosis

Exposure history and physical examination is usually sufficient to make the diagnosis. If patch testing is needed, a 0.1% ethanol extract of the Grevillea flower in petrolatum can be used [41].

Cross reactions

Due to structural similarity between resorcinols and urushiol, there is a high rate of cross- reactivity to *toxicodendron species* in patients sensitized to proteaceae plants.

Primulaceae Family

Members of the primulaceae family include many species of primrose such as the fairy primrose (*P. malacoides*), the Chinese primrose (*P. sinensis*) and the common primrose (*P. vulgaris*). They typically grow in cooler or mountainous regions in the Northern Hemisphere [9]. Originally native to China, primrose species were exported to England and to a lesser degree to America in the 1880s [41]. Most primrose are low- growing perennial herbs with colorful flowers. Due to the beauty of the flowers, primrose is commonly planted for its ornamental value in gardens and greenhouses.

Primulaceae- induced allergic contact dermatitis

Primrose species not only cause the typical linearly arranged ACD but can also cause facial dermatitis or hand dermatitis that is worse on the dominant hand [41]. Reports of primulaceae-induced ACD mimicking lichen planus, erythema multiforme or vitiligo have also been reported [1, 27, 2]. It can also cause airborne contact dermatitis when the allergen is released in pollen [14].

The main allergen is primin (2-methoxy-6-*n*-pentyl-*p*-benzoquinone). Primin is created from its precursor miconidin via oxidation, and resides in the terminal cells of microscopic hairs on the leaves, stems and flowers. Levels of primin within individual plants are highly varied and depend on specific species, season, amount of sunlight and cultivation method. Allergenicitiy is generally higher in warmer months and can be reduced by over-watering the plant [41, 29]. Interestingly, a primin deficient variant of *P. obconica* Hanse has been introduced in Europe and has led to decreased incidence of primulaeceae- induced ACD.

Diagnosis

While history and clinical examination is often enough to make the diagnosis, patch testing may aid in confirming the diagnosis. Primin in 0.01% petrolatum is available in European patch test series [41, 18].

Rutaceae Family

The rutaceae family includes numerous species found in tropical or temperate climates in Africa and Australia. However, certain members of the rutaceae family are widely cultivated including the citrus genus. Plants within the citrus genus that can cause ACD include lemon (*Citrus limon*), orange (*Citrus sinensis*) and bergamot (*Citrus aurantium*) [41]. Products from citrus genus are not only widely-found in the food industry, but also in the creation of aromatic oils, perfumes, soaps and cosmetics.

Rutaceae- induced allergic contact dermatitis

ACD due to rutaceae in its natural form is uncommon but can occur as hand dermatitis in those who habitually handle the plants. More commonly, patients become sensitized to these allergens present in cosmetic and personal care products containing citrus derivatives. Beauticians and those working with citrus-containing cosmeceuticals are at increased risk [26]. Sensitizers of citrus fruits in the rutaceae family include geraniol, citral and D-limonene [10]. The exact mechanism of sensitization is not known.

Diagnosis

Thorough exposure history, including history of use of fragrances, essential oils, soaps and cosmetics, may raise suspicion for citrus-induced ACD. Patch testing could help confirm the diagnosis, although no single standardized patch test allergen exists. Limonene is commercially available in 3% petrolatum for patch testing [41].

Alliaceae Family

The allium genus is a main genus within the alliaceae family. Members of this genus include common food crops including onion (*Allium cepa*), garlic (*A. sativum*), chive (*A. Schoenoprasum*) and leek (*A. porrum*). Other species within this family are grown as ornamental border plants. In general members of this species can be identified by their six-petalled flowers and soft linear leaves with a pungent garlicky aroma [5].

Alliaceae- induced allergic contact dermatitis

Alliaceae- induced ACD typically presents as fingertip dermatitis in patients with a history of handling plants of this family. Unlike other forms of hand ACD, alliaceae- induced ACD can involve fingertips of the index and middle fingers of the nondominant hand as well as the thumb of the dominant hand. This pattern of distribution is due to the fact that the bulb is held between the thumb and index or middle finger of the non-dominant hand while the knife is held in the dominant hand while cutting [41]. An eczematous eruption involving the palms is also possible. Alliaceae species have also been reported to cause a pemphigus-vulgaris like eruption, cheilitis and systemic contact dermatitis [15, 25, 38].

The sensitizing agent present in alliaceae species is diallyl disulfide which is present in the sap of the plant. The allergenic sap is released when any part of the plant is damaged.

Diagnosis

Comprehensive exposure history is critical in making the diagnosis. Patch testing can help confirm the diagnosis. The recommended testing allergen is 1% diallyl disulfide in petrolatum [23].

Cross Reaction

Due to structural similarities between the causative allergens, patients who are sensitized to one member of the family may cross react to another member [3].

Brassicaceae Family

The brassicaceae family, formerly known as the cruciferae family, is a family of flowering plants which includes many vegetables. Well- known members of this family include cabbage (*Brassica oleracea*), cauliflower (*B. oleracea var. botrytis*), turnip (*B. campestris*), mustard (*B. nigra*) radish (*Raphanus sativus*), and horseradish (*Armoracia rusticana*). Considered a relative of the mustard family is the *Capparaceae* family which includes the caper bush (*Capparis spinosa*). The caper bush, is a shrub with gray oval leaves and white-pink flowers with prominent stamens. The bud and fruit of the caper bush, colloquially referred to as capers, are often consumed in the pickled form [41].

Brassiaceae- induced allergic contact dermatitis

ACD due to this species is most commonly seen in food handlers and often presents with eczematous or vesiculobullous dermatitis on the hands. The allergen is isothiocyanate which is also a potent irritant. As a result, ICD is more common than ACD.

Diagnosis

Exposure history is key to making the diagnosis. Careful examination and elicitation of exposure timeline may help to differentiate between ICD and ACD [33].

Parmeliaceae Family

Foliose lichens are complex organisms which result from the symbiotic relationship between fungi and algae or cyanobacteria [6]. Parmelia is the largest genus of foliose lichens, which are simple, slow-growing plants that typically grow on rock, tree bark or wood. They have greenish- or bluish-gray leathery leaf- like structures, with a black underside [8]. Colloquial names for these plants include crottle and skull lichen.

Parmelia- induced allergic contact dermatitis

ACD due to lichens presents most often in patients with outdoor exposures. However, some lichens are used in indoor flower arrangements or Christmas decorations. Eczematous or vesiculobullous lesions develop on exposed skin, typically on the hands/upper extremities as a result of touching or carrying wood or rocks on which lichens have grown. Airborne contact dermatitis is also possible [28]. Allergens responsible for lichen-induced ACD include usinic acid, atranorin and evernic acid.

Diagnosis

A history of lichen exposure should raise suspicion for lichen- induced ACD. Patch testing can help confirm the diagnosis. Usinic acid, evernic acid and atranorin are available for patch testing.

Araliaceae Family

The araliaceae family is comprised mostly of shrubs and trees native to tropical climates; some species have become popular as houseplants as well. One of the most well-known species belonging to this family is common ivy (*Hedera helix*), an evergreen plant that climbs over rocks, trees, walls and other structures (Fig. 5).

Araliaceae- induced allergic contact dermatitis

Araliaceae- induced ACD presents similarly to other ACD with eczematous or vesiculobullous eruptions on exposed sites such as the hands and forearms. Face, neck or widespread involvement is also possible. Asthma induced by *H. helix* has also been reported [20, 53].

The allergens are falcarinol and didehydrofalcarinol which are present in the roots, stems and leaves.

Diagnosis

Exposure history will aid in making the diagnosis. Patch testing with falcarinol and didehydrofalcarinol in petrolatum is possible. Using plant material itself or plant extract to patch test is of low utility due to high false positive rates, possibly due to its irritating nature [41].

Cross reactions

Patients sensitized to plants of the araliaceae family may cross-react with *Daucus carota*, commonly known as carrot. The carrot is a common root vegetable cultivated for culinary use and contains falcarinol. Falcarinol is also found in celery (*Apium graveolens*) [41, 34].

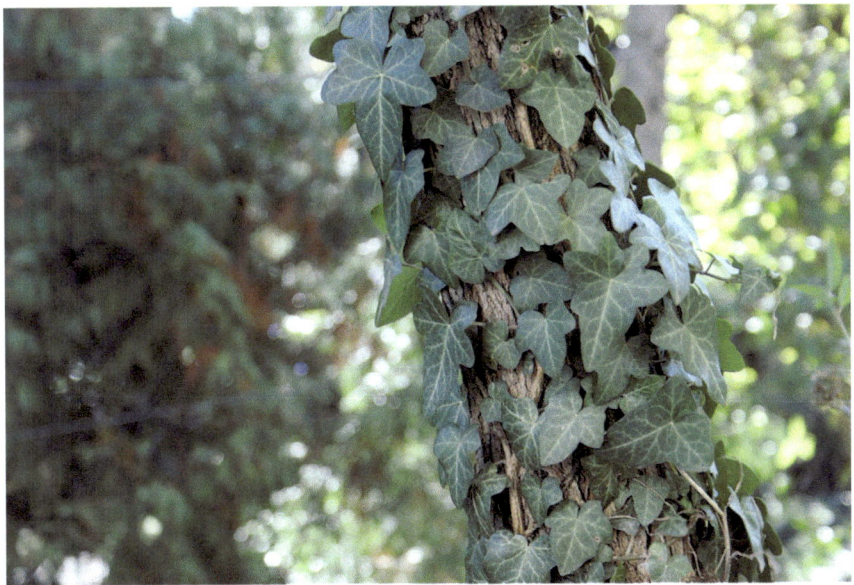

Fig. 5 *Hedera helix* (common ivy), is a member of the *Araliaceae* family. Photo courtesy of: chery (https://commons.wikimedia.org/wiki/File:Hedera_helix_clinging.jpg), "Hedera helix clinging", marked as public domain, more details on Wikimedia Commons: https://commons.wikimedia.org/wiki/Template:PD-self

Prevention of Allergic Contact Dermatitis to Plants

Avoiding contact with plants known to cause ACD is the most effective way to prevent sensitization. If complete avoidance is not possible, protective clothing should be worn. However, plant resin can stay on clothing for several days after exposure. As a result, protective clothing should be washed in warm soapy water. If contact is made with a culprit allergen, the exposed skin should be washed with mild soap and warm water as soon as possible. If repeat exposure is likely, patients may benefit from application of a barrier cream containing bentoquatam [42]. Bentoquatam, an organoclay compound, has been shown to prevent or diminish contact dermatitis due to *Toxicodendron species* [31]. Outdoor pets who come into contact with culprit plants may carry the allergens for several days and transfer them to humans upon contact. Therefore, care should be taken to wash these animals thoroughly after exposure.

Management of Allergic Contact Dermatitis to Plants

Symptoms of allergic contact dermatitis are most effectively managed with corticosteroids. For localized disease, topical steroids are appropriate. Ultra-potent topical steroids are thought to be most effective and are safe for short- term use, even under occlusion. Patients with severe or generalized ACD may benefit from an oral corticosteroid taper, starting at 1 mg/kg/day. A taper course lasting 14–21 days is recommended, as too short of a course typically results in a rebound dermatitis. Intramuscular or intralesional injections of corticosteroids could also be considered.

Symptomatic management of ACD due to plants may also involve other topical therapies such as calamine lotion, which may be soothing, or topical astringents, which may help dry up the vesicobullous lesions and associated drainage. Oral antihistamines may be beneficial in reducing itch. Secondary infection should be treated with appropriate topical or oral antibiotics.

Conclusion

Many plant species can cause ACD. Frequent handlers of these plants are at increased risk for sensitization. Common presentations of plants induced ACD include well demarcated eczematous or vesicobullous eruption or fissured plaques at sites of exposure. Diagnosis is made based on history and physical examination. Patch testing may be needed in confirmation of the diagnosis.

References

1. Angelini DB. Erythema multiforme-like contact dermatitis from primin. Contact Dermat. 2008;174–176.
2. Bhushan M, Beck MH. Allergic contact dermatitis from primula presenting as vitiligo. Contact Dermat. 2007;292–293.
3. Bleumink EDH. Allergic contact dermatitis to garlic. Br J Dermatol. 1972;6–9.
4. Bressette DK. *Pacific poison oak, Toxicodendron diversilobum* (2017, January 2). Retrieved from Native Plants PNW: https://www.nativeplantspnw.com/poison-oak-toxicodendron-diversilobum/.
5. Brittanica TE. Allium. Encycl Brittanica. (n.d.).
6. Brittanica TE. Lichen. Encycl Brittanica. (n.d.).
7. Brittanica TE. Liliaceae. Encycl Brittanica.
8. Brittanica TE. Parmelia. Encycl Brittanica. (n.d.).
9. Brittanica TE. Primrose. Encycl Brittanica.
10. Cardullo AC, Ruszkowski AM, DeLeo VA. Allergic contact dermatitis resulting from sensitivity to citrus peel, geraniol, and citral. J Am Acad Dermatol. 1989;395–97.
11. Chadwick M, Trewin H, Gawthrop F, Wagstaff C. Sesquiterpenoids lactones: benefits to plants and people. Int J Mol Sci. 2013;12780–805.
12. Chastant LR. Black-spot poison ivy, a report of 3 cases with clinicopathologic correlation. JAAD Case Rep. 2018;140–42.
13. Christen M, Mowad BA. Allergic contact dermatitis: patient diagnosis and evaluation. J Am Acad Dermatol. 2016;74. (Danville, PA).
14. Christensen LP, Larsen E. Direct emission of the allergen primin from intact Primula obconica plants. Contact Dermat. 2000;149–53.

15. Ekeowaanderson AL, Shergill B, Goldsmith P. Allergic contact cheilitis to garlic. Contact Dermat. 2007;174–175.
16. Fisher A. Fischer's contact dermatitis. Baltimore, MD: Williams & Wilkins; 1995.
17. Forest Serivce, Department of Agriculture. Toxicodendron radicans; 2019. Retrieved from Fire Effects Information System.
18. Fregert S, Hjorth N, Schulz KH. Patch testing with synthetic primin in persons sensitive to primula obconica. JAMA Dermatol.1968
19. Gladman AC. Toxicodendron dermatitis: poison ivy, oak and sumac. Wilderness Environ Med. 2006;17(2):120–8.
20. Hannu T, Kauppi P, Tuppurainen M, Piirilä P. Occupational asthma to ivy (Hedera helix). Allergy. 2008;482–483.
21. Hausen BM, Prater E, Schubert H. The sensitizing capacity of Alstroemeria cultivars in man and guinea pig. Remarks on the occurrence, quantity and irritant and sensitizing potency of their constituents tuliposide A and tulipalin A (alpha-methylene-gamma-butyrol-actone). Contact Dermat. 1983;46–54.
22. Hausen B. Allergenic hardwoods. In: Javier Avalos HM, editor. Dermatologic botany. CRC Press; 1999.
23. Hjorth N, Roed-Petersen J. Occupational protein contact dermatitis in food handlers. Contact Dermat. 1976;28–42.
24. Hjorth N, Wilkinson DS. Contact dermatitis IV. Tulip fingers, hyacinth itch and lily rash. British J Dermatol. 1969;696–98.
25. Jappe U, Bonnekoh B, Hausen BM, Gollnick H. Garlic-related dermatoses: case report and review of the literature. Contact Dermat. 1999;37–39.
26. Johnston PD. An outbreak of allergic contact dermatitis caused by citral in beauticians working in a health spa. Contact Dermat. 2014;377–79.
27. Lapière K, Matthieu L, Meuleman L, Lambert J. Primula dermatitis mimicking lichen planus. Contact Dermat. 2001;199.
28. Lorenzi SG. Airborne contact dermatitis from atranorin. Contact Dermat. 1995
29. Lovell CG. Contact dermatitis due to hardy primula species and their cultivars. Contact Dermat. 2008;23–29.
30. Luz S, Fonacier JM. Allergic contact dermatitis. Ann Allergy Asthma Immunol. 2014;9–12.
31. Marks JG Jr, Fowler JF Jr, Sheretz EF, Rietschel RL. Prevention of poison ivy and poison oak allergic contact dermatitis by quaternium-18 bentonite. J Am Acad Dermatol. 1995;33(2 Pt 1):212–6. PubMed PMID: 7622647.
32. McCall BP. Incidence rates, costs, severity and work-related factors of occupational dermatitis. JAMA Dermatol. 2005;713–718.
33. Mitchell J. Contact dermatitis from plants of the caper family. Capparidaceae. Effects on the skin of some plants which yield isothiocyanates. British J Dermatol. 1974;13–20.
34. Murdoch SR, Dempster J. Allergic contact dermatitis from carrot. Contact Dermat. 2000;236.
35. Ohio State University, College of Food, Agricultural, and Environmental Sciences. Ohio Perennial and Biennial Weed Guide; 2019.
36. Paulsen E, Christensen LP, Andersen KE. Possible cross-reactivity between para-phenylenediamine and sesquiterpene lactones. Contact Dermat. 2008;120–122.
37. Paulsen E, Andersen KE, Hausen BM Sensitization and cross-reaction patterns in Danish Compositae-allergic patients. Contact Dermat. 2001;197–204.
38. Pereira F, Hatia M, Cardoso J. Systemic contact dermatitis from diallyl disulfide. Contact Dermat. 2002;124.
39. Powell S. Contact dermatitis from rhus verniciflua- further evidence concerning the hazard of domestic planting. Arboric J. 1987;165–168.
40. Rademaker JG. Allergic contact dermatitis from exposure to Grevillea robusta in New Zealand. Australas J Dermatol. 2009;125–128.

41. Rozas-Muñoz E, Lepoittevin JP, Pujol RM, Giménez-Arnau A. Allergic contact dermatitis to plants: understanding the chemistry will help our diagnostic approach. Actas Dermo-Sifiliogr. 2012;103.
42. Scott MJ, Heumann MA, DeBruyckere DM, Brundage TW, Kohn MA. The feasibility of using skin protectant products and education to prevent poison oak. Wilderness Environ Med. 2002;13(3):206–8. PubMed PMID: 12353598.
43. Semalty M. Semecarpus anacardium Linn.: A review. Pharmacogn Rev. 2010;88–94.
44. Skolmen RG. Silk-Oak (n.d.). Retrieved from https://www.srs.fs.usda.gov.
45. The Editors of Encyclopaedia Brittanica. Asteraceae. Encycl Brittanica.
46. United States Department of Agriculture. *Anacardium occidentale*; 2019. Retrieved from Plants database.
47. United States Department of Agriculture. Plant Guide: Mango; 2004. Retrieved from Natural Resources Conservation Service.
48. United States Department of Agriculture. *Schinus terebinthifolius Raddi*; 2019. Retrieved from Plants database.
49. United States Department of Agriculture. *Toxicodendron vernix*; 2019. Retrieved from Plant Database.
50. University of Florida Institute of Food and Agricultural Sciences. *Schinus terebinthifolius*; 2019. Retrieved from http://www.plants.ifas.ufl.edu/wp-content/uploads/files/caip/reco_cards/schter.pdf.
51. US Fish and Wildlife Service. Poisonous Plants: Poison Ivy, Sumac, and Oak. Shiawassee National Wildlife Refuge.
52. Wilkinson SM, Pollock B. Patch test sensitization after use of Compositae mix. Contact Dermat. 1999;277–8.
53. Yesudian PD, Franks A. Contact dermatitis from Hedera helix in a husband and wife. Contact Dermat. 2002;125–126.

Arachnida: Spiders and Scorpions

Paul A. Regan, Galen T. Foulke and Elizabeth J. Usedom

Spiders

Paul A. Regan and Galen T. Foulke

Introduction

Definitive diagnosis of spider bites is a point of contention for researchers and medical professionals alike. In the United States, roughly 60 different species of spiders have been implicated in human bites and more than 100,000 bites are reported yearly [1, 2]. However, in the majority of cases, a spider bite is only presumed, as a bite is rarely witnessed or a spider captured. Spider bites are an exceedingly rare cause of significant morbidity and mortality. Several spiders, however, are clinically important and are a recognized source of morbidity and potentially life-threatening complications.

Spiders are members of the arthropod phylum and comprise the largest order (Araneae) within the class of arachnids, which also includes scorpions, ticks, and mites [3]. Scorpions are discussed later in this chapter. Ticks and mites are

P. A. Regan · G. T. Foulke (✉)
Department of Dermatology, Penn State Health Milton S. Hershey Medical Center, Hershey, PA, USA
e-mail: galenfoulke@gmail.com; gfoulke@pennstatehealth.psu.edu

P. A. Regan
e-mail: pregan@pennstatehealth.psu.edu

E. J. Usedom
Department of Dermatology, Wright State University Boonshoft School of Medicine, Dayton, OH, USA
e-mail: ejusedom@gmail.com

© Springer Nature Switzerland AG 2020
J. Trevino and A. Y-Y. Chen (eds.), *Dermatological Manual of Outdoor Hazards*,
https://doi.org/10.1007/978-3-030-37782-3_6

discussed in Chaps. 8 and 9, respectively. More than 40,000 distinct species of spiders inhabit varied ecological systems throughout the world. Anatomically, spiders have eight legs connected to a body composed of two segments, the cephalothorax and the abdomen. The cephalothorax is primarily responsible for food ingestion and neurological function, while the abdomen contains structures that perform digestion, circulation, reproduction, and silk production. The typical spider ranges from 2-10 mm in body length, with males tending to be smaller than females. Almost all spiders are carnivorous, capturing their insect prey in webs or on the ground. They employ sharp fangs at the ends of mouth appendages, called chelicerae, to bite and envenomate their prey. While many spiders are venomous, the fangs of most spiders lack the length or strength necessary to penetrate human skin and inject venom [4]. As a result, most spider bites cause minimal local or systemic effects.

Two genera of spiders in the United States are widely accepted as being medically important: the *Loxosceles*, or recluse spiders, and the *Latrodectus*, or widow spiders. Bites from other spiders, such as hobo spiders and tarantulas, have been reported but are considered to be of minimal medical seriousness. This section seeks to describe the medically significant spiders in the United States as well as summarize the diagnostic and treatment approaches to spider bites.

Clinical Findings and Diagnosis

The clinical findings associated with spider bites vary greatly. Symptomatic bites are mainly benign, causing only mild, temporary cutaneous changes [4]. In the cases where a dermal reaction occurs, most present as a single, local lesion. Papules, plaques, pustules, wheals, and ulcers have all been described. A hypersensitivity reaction, either from the bite itself or from contact with the spider, may produce papular urticaria [5]. Necrotic lesions, termed necrotic arachnidism, can result from the bites of certain spiders and will be discussed below [6]. Systemic effects, such as fever, chills, nausea, vomiting, arthralgias, muscle weakness, and hematologic abnormalities, are possible from envenoming bites, and they tend to be characteristic of certain species (see below). Although pain and discomfort at the site of the bite are common, some bites may go unnoticed. The affected area may become pruritic and erythematous. Puncture marks from fangs may or may not be visible [4]. The most common location of spider bites is the distal extremities, particularly the hands [6].

The diagnosis of a spider bite can be challenging, but it should be considered in the setting of a pustular or necrotic lesion of unknown origin [4]. Oftentimes, the spider is never seen or recovered for identification [1]. The differential diagnosis of a spider bite is broad (Fig. 1). The typical skin manifestations resulting from spider bites closely resemble those of other dermatologic and systemic conditions, particularly folliculitis or furunculosis [6]. The primary focus should be placed on ruling out an infectious etiology, which is the most likely diagnosis when a spider bite is considered [7].

Infectious	Exposures	Vascular	Other
Furuncle	Tick	Venous stasis ulcer	Pyoderma gangrenosum
Folliculitis	Millipede	Diabetic ulcer	Erythema nodosum
Cellulitis	Centipede	Vasculitis	Nonmelanoma skin cancer
Herpes simplex	Scorpion		Contact dermatitis
Dermatomycosis	Mosquito		
Lyme disease	Bee		
Sporotrichosis	Wasp		
Cutaneous anthrax			
Tularemia			
Cat scratch disease			

Fig. 1 Differential diagnosis of a spider bite

When a spider bite is definitively witnessed and the spider is identified, then the diagnosis can be reasonably confirmed. Otherwise, the diagnosis of a spider bite is made clinically by ruling out other potential etiologies. Despite the high incidence of reported spider bites, clinicians should undertake a careful consideration of alternative diagnoses as there is usually a more likely explanation underlying the patient's presentation.

Spiders

The two main spiders of medical importance in the United States are the brown recluse spider (*Loxosceles reclusa*) and the black widow spider (*Latrodectus mactans*). Several other spiders that are known to bite humans but are exceedingly unlikely to cause significant morbidity and mortality will also be discussed briefly.

Brown Recluse (Loxosceles reclusa)

Epidemiology The brown recluse spider is found in the Southeast and Midwest United States [4]. The spider resides in warm, dark places such as attics, closets, and under rocks and woodpiles. It has a distinctive violin- or fiddle-shaped marking on the dorsal aspect of the cephalothorax (Fig. 2) [1]. The length of the female brown recluse spider measures between 8-15 mm. Brown recluse spiders are shy and do not bite humans unless threatened or provoked [7]. Bites can produce a necrotic ulcerating lesion but are almost never life-threatening. They occur most frequently in the spring and summer months.

Signs and Symptoms The bite from a brown recluse spider may cause a localized, minor stinging or burning pain, or may be painless [4]. The initial wound presents as transient erythema with the formation of a single papule, pustule, or vesicle [8]. Cutaneous lesions that are large, numerous, chronic, swollen, or exudative are unlikely to be from the bite of a brown recluse spider [9]. The classic

Fig. 2 Brown recluse spider
(Reprinted by permission
from Springer Nature:
Springer; *Loxosceles* spiders
by Malaque et al. [20])

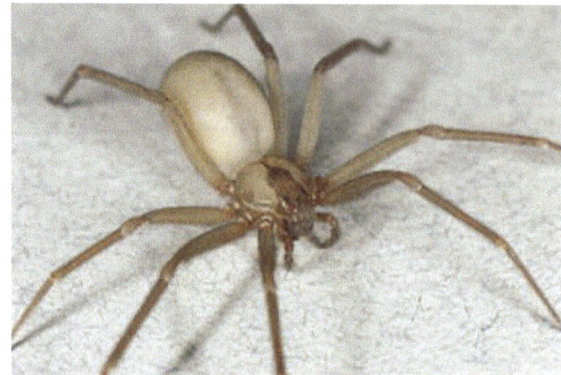

Fig. 3 a "Red, white, and
blue" sign: an erythematous
ring surrounding a central
violaceous area. **b** Necrotic
arachnidism: necrosis with
eschar formation (Reprinted
by permission from Springer
Nature: Springer; Brown
recluse spider bite by Gloster
et al. [21])

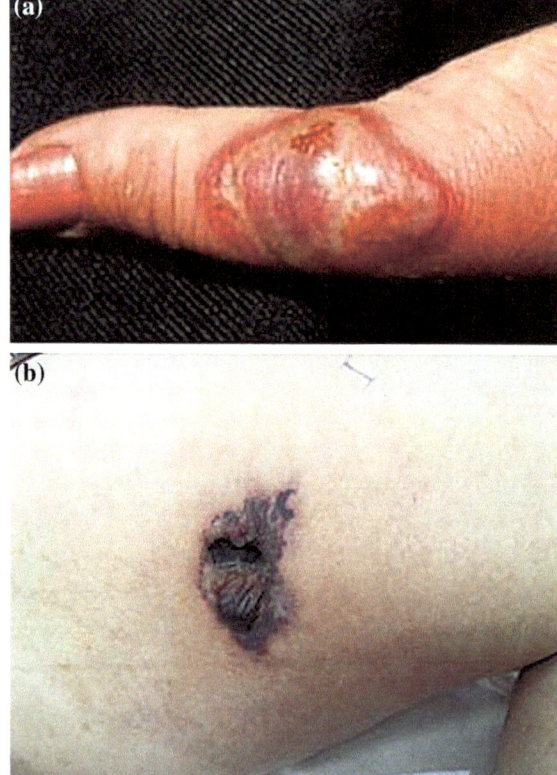

clinical description of a brown recluse bite is known as the "red, white, and blue"
sign: a central violaceous area that becomes surrounded by a blanching halo and
an erythematous border (Fig. 3a) [8]. Necrosis develops in a minority of the cases
in the days following the bite (Fig. 3b). It is mediated by the main component

of brown recluse venom, sphingomyelinase D, which induces a proinflammatory response and local tissue damage. Hyaluronidase, another component of the recluse's venom, is thought to facilitate the spread of local erythema and necrosis [10]. Necrotic ulcers can take months to heal and can result in significant scarring [11]. Systemic reactions do occur but are often mild and involve nonspecific constitutional symptoms within the first 72 hours [6].

Treatment Initial treatment should include irrigation and cleansing of the wound site as well as application of ice or cold compresses [8]. Tetanus prophylaxis should be considered. Pain control can often be achieved with mild analgesics (acetaminophen or ibuprofen) [5]. Early signs of necrotic arachnidism or systemic symptoms may necessitate hospitalization. Wound care involves debridement of necrotic tissue and eschar [11]. Hyperbaric oxygenation, intralesional corticosteroids, and dapsone have all been tried to slow down the expansion of necrosis, but their effectiveness is unproven [11, 12]. Antibiotic therapy may be indicated to prevent secondary bacterial infection. A *Loxosceles* antivenom is used in South America but is not currently available in the United States [13].

Black Widow (*Latrodectus mactans*)

Epidemiology Though five species of widow spiders are found in the United States, the black widow spider, or *Latrodectus mactans*, is the most medically relevant. The black widow inhabits every state in the country but is more prevalent in the southern and western states [1]. It builds webs in dry, warm areas in both indoor and outdoor environments, such as the corner of a shed or garage or underneath a woodpile. The spider can be identified by its shiny black or dark gray color and the red/orange hourglass-shaped marking on the ventral side of its abdomen (Fig. 4). Female black widow spiders can grow up to 10 mm in body length [3].

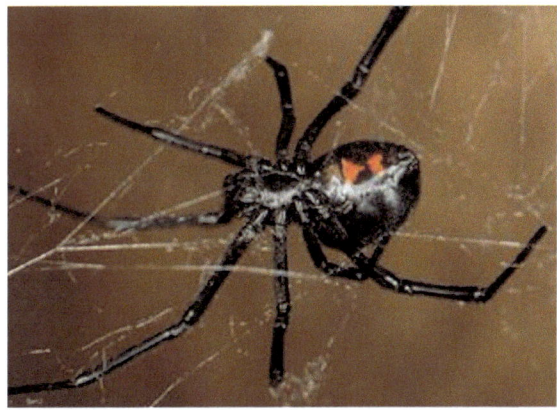

Fig. 4 Black widow spider (Reprinted by permission from Springer Nature: Springer; Envenomations by widow, recluse, and medically implicated spiders by Vetter et al. [22])

Fig. 5 Black widow
spider bite demonstrating
localized erythema without
dermal damage (Reprinted
by permission from
Springer Nature: Springer;
Envenomations by widow,
recluse, and medically
implicated spiders by Vetter
et al. [22])

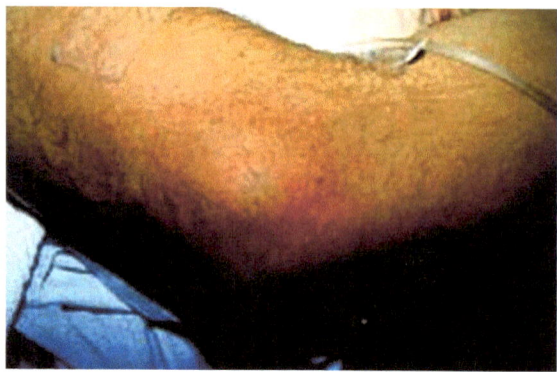

Black widow spiders are passive and tend to bite humans only when provoked [8]. Bites can be serious but seldom result in death [4].

Signs and Symptoms The initial manifestation of a black widow spider bite is usually mild pain and localized erythema at the bite site (Fig. 5) [4]. The surrounding skin can become urticarial or cyanotic [5]. If the skin was punctured, two small fang marks may be visible [1]. Necrosis is not seen in black widow spider bites [13]. Envenomation produces localized piloerection, sweating, and paresthesias around the bite site [14]. Systemic toxicity is the result of its venom, α-latrotoxin, which is a neurotoxin [8]. The toxin promotes presynaptic release of autonomic neurotransmitters at neuromuscular junctions and nerve endings, resulting in muscle spasm, back pain, and abdominal rigidity that mimics an acute abdomen. Other nonspecific symptoms such as fever, nausea, and headache may be present [7]. These systemic symptoms most often occur within 30 minutes to two hours of the bite. Both local and systemic manifestations resolve over the course of a few days.

Treatment In mild cases, pain can be relieved with a mild analgesic (acetaminophen or ibuprofen) [4]. Local wound care, including irrigation, cleansing, and ice application, should be performed [7]. Tetanus prophylaxis should also be administered if indicated. Hospitalization should be considered for young children, pregnant women, and the elderly, as they are more likely to experience severe systemic reactions [8, 11]. In severe cases, an opioid analgesic is combined with a muscle relaxant to combat pain and muscle spasms [8]. Calcium gluconate was used for this purpose in the past but is no longer recommended as narcotics and benzodiazepines are more effective [15]. *Latrodectus* antivenin can be used when systemic toxicity occurs, but it can cause serious allergic reactions [14].

Others

Hobo (*Eratigena agrestis*) The hobo spider resides in the Pacific northwest United States [1]. It is a larger spider with a body length of 10-15 mm and has a brown color with a distinctive herringbone stripe on its abdomen. It constructs webs in basements, wood piles, and gardens [7]. Unlike the *Latrodectus* and *Loxosceles* species, where the female spider is larger and more dangerous to humans, the male hobo spider is more venomous and is implicated in more bites than the female. The spider has been a suspected cause of necrotic arachnidism in the Pacific northwest states, but a lack of conclusive evidence remains [16]. Bites from the hobo spider are generally painless [8]. The area becomes indurated with surrounding erythema, which progresses to vesicle and blister formation [7]. The most common systemic symptoms include headache, nausea, fatigue, and temporary memory impairment [5]. Although rarely reported, aplastic anemia is the most serious potential consequence [17]. Bite sites typically heal spontaneously over weeks to months and treatment is symptom-directed [7].

Tarantula (*Theraphosidae*) The majority of tarantulas in the United States are found in burrows and under rocks in the desert regions of the Southwest [4]. Some species are also kept as household pets [8]. Tarantulas are among the world's largest spiders and are often hairy and colorful (Fig. 6). They rarely inflict envenoming bites in humans. When they do occur, bites cause a minor stinging pain and a local inflammatory reaction. There are no systemic symptoms [11]. Tarantulas have urticating hairs on their dorsal abdomen that can be launched toward aggressors as a defense mechanism. The hairs, which are chitinous projections of the spider's exoskeleton, cause a pruritic reaction if they penetrate human skin [10]. If the hairs lodge in the cornea of the eye, an inflammatory reaction called ophthalmia nodosa can ensue, which necessitates immediate referral to an ophthalmologist [18]. Treatment of bites is focused on wound cleansing, analgesia, and tetanus prophylaxis [11]. In the case of pruritic eruption from urticating hairs, antihistamines and topical corticosteroids are used [8].

Wolf spiders (*Lycosa*), jumping spiders (*Phiddipus*), and running spiders (*Liocranoides*) All of these spiders have been implicated in human bites with minimal clinical significance [1]. Bites can be treated symptomatically and with local wound care, as well as mild analgesics if needed.

Fig. 6 Tarantula spider (Reprinted by permission from Springer Nature: Springer; Behavior and biology of mygalomorphae by Pérez-Miles et al. [23])

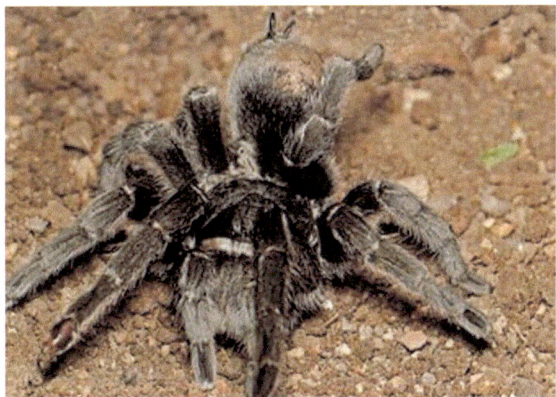

Conclusion

The two most medically important spiders in the United States are the brown recluse spider (*Loxosceles reclusa*) and black widow spider (*Latrodectus mactans*). Bites from these spiders can rarely be life-threatening. Bites from other spiders, such as the hobo spider, tarantula, or wolf spider, tend to be clinically minor. The differential diagnosis of spider bites is broad and includes other skin and soft tissue infections, bites and stings from other arthropods, and other causes of cutaneous ulceration. Unless the spider bite is witnessed, there are no diagnostic confirmatory tests. Treatment involves local wound care, pain control, and monitoring of systemic toxicity, with the additional considerations of tetanus and antibiotic prophylaxis. Spider bites can be prevented by wearing protective clothing and using insect repellent (N,N-diethyl-3-methylbenzamide (DEET)) when in wooded areas [19].

Scorpions

Elizabeth J. Usedom

Introduction

Worldwide, there are more than 1 million documented cases of scorpion envenomation with over 3,000 cases resulting in death [24, 25]. In the United States, only approximately 15 deaths from scorpion envenomation have been documented from 1979 to 2015 [26]. The vast majority of stings result in localized pain or minimal systemic symptoms. However, severe systemic symptoms are a major cause of morbidity and mortality. Scorpions stings inject an α-toxin which produces a neurotoxic excitation syndrome.

There are six families of scorpions; scorpions in the Buthidae family are the cause of the majority of clinically significant stings. The main exception is *Hemiscorpius lepturus*, endemic to Iran, belonging to the Hemiscorpiidae family, which causes a cytotoxic syndrome with overt cutaneous findings (erythema, purpura, bullae, ulcers, necrosis) in addition to neurotoxic symptoms [27]. There are numerous genera of scorpions within the Buthidae family throughout the world. The greatest number of stings worldwide occur in Brazil and Venezuela due to scorpions in the Tityinae subfamily of Buthidae. Notably, *Tityus serrulatus* has one of the most potent venoms and affects all anatomic systems. The well-known adverse effect of acute pancreatitis due to scorpion envenomation is caused by either scorpions in the Tityinae subfamily in Brazil or *Leiurus quinquestriatus* in the Middle East [24, 28]. Scorpions causing clinically significant morbidity in the United States belong to the genus Centruroides [5].

Scorpions have two major body segments, the prosoma and opithosoma [29]. The prosoma is considered the head of the scorpion with median and lateral eyes, carapace, chelicera (mouth), and pedipalps (claws or pincers) used for grasping prey. The opithosoma is comprised of the mesosoma (body) and metosoma (tail). The tail is curved with a distal bulbous sac called the vesicle and terminates with a stinger used to incapacitate its prey. Scorpions have eight legs in addition to the pedipalps and tail and range from 1 to 20 cm in length. Venomous scorpions in family Buthidae can be differentiated from nonvenomous scorpions with their triangular-shaped sternum, smaller pincers, thinner bodies, and thicker tails. Scorpions are nocturnal creatures, hiding during the day to avoid higher temperatures or sunlight. They are often found under rocks, wood, or anything on the ground. Some may burrow into the ground, while others have the ability to climb trees or walls. Scorpions are shy and will only sting in defense when threatened [29].

Of the Centruroides genus, there are two medically important scorpions in the United States: the Arizona bark scorpion (*Centruroides exilicauda* or *sculpturatus*) and striped bark scorpion (*C. vittatus*). Other scorpions in the Centuroides genus, all found in Mexico, Central America, and part of the Southwest United States, cause a similar constellation of symptoms as the Arizona bark scorpion and include the Mexican scorpions (*C. noxious, C. limpidus*) and Durango bark scorpion (*C. suffusus*). This section describes these medically relevant scorpions in the United States and describes the clinical presentation and treatment of scorpion envenomation.

Clinical Findings and Diagnosis

Scorpion envenomation in the United States causes either localized pain with minimal cutaneous findings or systemic symptoms resulting from the neurotoxic excitation syndrome from hematologic dissemination of the α-toxin in scorpion venom [24, 27]. Stings from scorpions in the United States often present with few if any cutaneous findings. Upon the initial sting, there is immediate, sharp, burning pain with resultant numbness. The site of sting may be mildly evident and associated with local edema and erythema. Regional lymphadenopathy and muscle fasciculations may also occur. Centruroides predominately cause neuromuscular toxicity when systemic symptoms occur. The α-toxin causes autonomic excitation with the release of epinephrine and norepinephrine and other vasoactive proteins, neuropeptide Y and endothelin-1 [24]. Sympathetic effects are more pronounced than parasympathetic. The powerful neurotoxin can cause muscle spasticity and fasciculations, excessive salivation, nystagmus, visual/auditory disturbances, slurred speech, and respiratory distress due to uncoordinated neuromuscular activity. Other scorpions outside the United States cause more cardiovascular toxicity, but all stings from the more potent scorpions can result in the most dangerous effects: pulmonary edema and cardiogenic shock. Hypersensitivity reactions after striped bark scorpion envenomation have also been described [30]. It is important to note that scorpions outside the United States not related to the Centruroides genus may cause more pronounced cutaneous manifestations as previously mentioned.

Scorpion stings are typically identified by the patient as the sting results in immediate, severe pain and the scorpion is large enough to be identified immediately. No specific diagnostic testing exists. All stings should be graded based on clinical effects to monitor for signs of progression and determine the appropriate treatment (Table 1) [24, 31].

Scorpions

The two scorpions of clinical importance in the United States are the Arizona bark scorpion (*C. exilicauda* or *sculpturatus*) and the striped bark scorpion (*C. vittatus*). Other scorpions within the United States are not known to cause clinically significant effects. The only exception is the Arizona striped-tail or devil scorpion (*Vaejovis spinigerus*), which may cause only local edema [26]. There are other scorpions causing disease outside the United States and have been briefly mentioned prior (Fig. 7).

Arizona Bark Scorpion (Centruroides exilicauda, Centruroides sculpturatus)

Epidemiology The Arizona bark scorpion is found in the Southeastern United States, especially in Arizona, as the name implies. Both names *C. exilicauda* and *C. sculpturatus* (previously *C. gertschi*) have been used interchangeably, but likely

Table 1 Clinical Grade of Scorpion Envenomation and Associated Treatment [24, 31]

Clinical grade	Clinical effects	Treatment
I. Local	Isolated local effects	Ice, analgesia, local anesthesia
II. Minor	Agitation, anxiety, confusion, hypertension, encephalopathy, hypothermia	Antivenom, oral benzodiazepines (BZP)
III. Major	CNS: acute paralysis, brain edema, ischemia on CT/MRI, coma Pulmonary: respiratory failure, pulmonary edema, cyanosis Cardiogenic: shock, hypotension, ventricular arrhythmias	Admission to ICU, antivenom, supportive care, BZP infusion
IV. Lethal	Multiple organ failure	Admission to ICU, supportive care, mechanical ventilation, BZP infusion

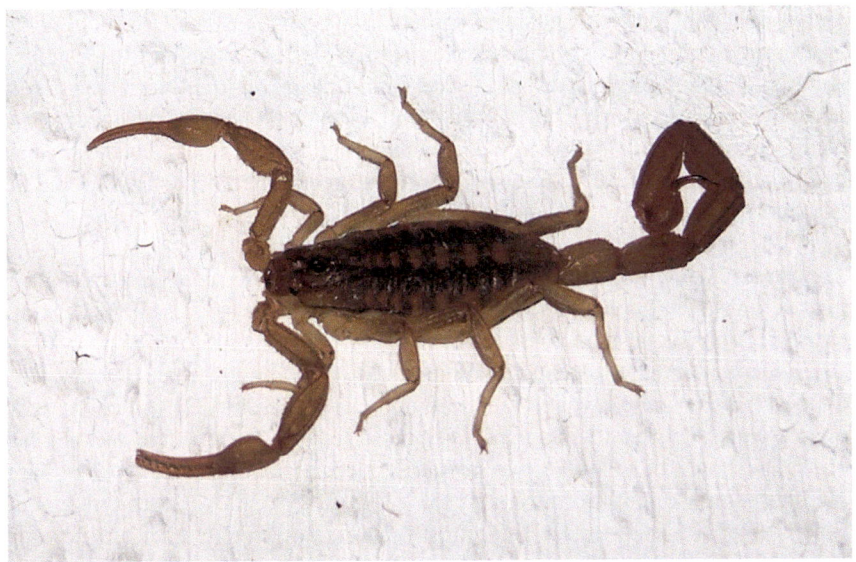

Fig. 7 Durango bark scorpion, *Centruroides suffuses*. Note the thin pincers, thin body, and thick tail indicative of venomous scorpions. By Drini (Pedro Sánchez). Credit: CC-BY-SA (2.5)+GFDL

represent two different species albeit very closely related. For the purposes of this section and in review of the literature, the species can be considered synonymous, causing the same medically relevant syndrome.

The Arizona bark scorpion is found in arid climates and prefers darker crevices, often under rocks or wood [5]. The majority of stings occur in the summer and early fall months when the temperature is higher, forcing the scorpion into cooler buildings. Stings are most frequent in the evening as the scorpion is most active at this time. As with other scorpions, the Arizona bark scorpion is shy and will only sting in defense to a threat. The scorpion has been found in many different colors, usually light in color, with longer pedipalps. A distinguishing feature is a spine, or tubercle, at the very base of the stinger. They can measure anywhere from 1.3 to 7.6 cm in length [5].

Signs and Symptoms The Arizona bark scorpion is responsible for the more severe and lethal cases in the United States, the vast majority of which occur in Arizona. The sting of the Arizona bark scorpion is very painful and typically presents with very limited cutaneous findings. The most common associated symptom is numbness [26]. Localized edema or erythema may result, but is not as frequently observed. Neurologic symptoms may become apparent within the hour after the sting and include muscle fasciculations, decreased fine-motor movement, excessive salivation, nystagmus, visual/auditory disturbances, slurred speech, and respiratory distress. Additional findings of autonomic excitation may also be apparent in the form of agitation, anxiety, and hypertension. Cardiopulmonary symptoms may manifest with increasing time from envenomation, especially in children. Clinical progression of envenomation in children younger than 2 years occurs on average within 14 minutes [32]. The most feared cardiopulmonary complications include pulmonary edema and cardiogenic shock. Death is usually due to respiratory or cardiovascular failure and most often occurs within the first 24 hours of a sting.

Treatment Patients presenting with only localized clinical symptoms may be treated with local application of ice and anesthetics if desired. Although the systemic neuromuscular symptoms are more common after Arizona bark scorpions envenomation, lethality is uncommon in adults. Children less than 10 years are at greatest risk for more severe systemic symptoms and death [32]. All children and infants with a scorpion sting, especially those likely caused by the Arizona bark scorpion, should be admitted to a pediatric intensive care unit for close monitoring and administration of antivenom [33]. The *Centruroides* (Scorpion) Immune F(ab′)2 Injection (trade name, Anascorp) is a safe antivenom with a very low incidence of adverse immune reactions. Anaphylactic reactions are very uncommon and serum sickness occurs in <1% of patients. Additionally, the serum sickness due to antivenom is self-limited and managed with antihistamines and steroids [34]. Earlier administration of antivenom has been shown to prevent progression and resolve clinical effects of envenomation quickly. As shown in Table 1, administration of antivenom should be standard with Grades II and III clinical presentation. Once antivenom is administered, resolution of neuromuscular symptoms typically occurs within 30 minutes to 4 hours [32, 33, 35]. It is important to note that antivenom is less effective once severe envenomation has occurred as the antivenom works to bind circulating toxins, that which have yet to establish system compromise [24].

Striped Bark Scorpion (Centruroides vittatus)

Epidemiology The striped bark scorpion is found in the Central United States, especially in Texas. It is the most common scorpion in the United States. They are found most often in dark crevices and may be found in homes. This species does not burrow but can climb; therefore, it may be found in attics in endemic regions [29]. Although the striped bark scorpion can tolerate a wide range of climatic conditions, they tend to avoid high temperatures by moving indoors during summer months, increasing the risk of human contact. The scorpion is usually yellowish-brown with longitudinal stripes on its mesosoma and its distinguishing variety of shapes on the carapace. They can measure up to 7 cm in length [29].

Signs and Symptoms The predominant symptom after a striped bark scorpion sting is significant localized pain [24]. Often the pain associated with the sting will be out of proportion to the clinical findings as the sting does not produce obvious cutaneous changes. These scorpions are not associated with systemic symptoms resulting from their toxin as it is much less potent than that of other scorpions in the genus. However, due to the high incidence of striped bark scorpion stings, there have been a number of documented hypersensitivity reactions, including urticaria, pruritus, flushing, angioedema, and other signs and symptoms of anaphylaxis [30]. These reactions are often confused with the neurological symptoms caused by other scorpions. Venom specific IgE can be identified in this subset of patients [30].

Treatment Due to the lack of systemic symptoms, these stings can be treated with local application of cold compresses. If local anesthetic is required due to severe pain, localized injection of lidocaine 2% or bupivacaine 0.5% without vasoconstrictors is preferred [27].

Conclusion

The most medically relevant scorpions in the United States are the Arizona bark scorpion (*C. exilicauda* or *sculpturatus*) and the striped bark scorpion (*C. vittatus*). Stings from these scorpions cause significant pain without overt cutaneous findings. The Arizona bark scorpion sting can be life-threatening. Most scorpion stings are witnessed, obviating the need for diagnostic testing. Clinical effects should be graded on a scale of I to IV, Grade I indicating local symptoms and Grade IV indicating multiple organ failure. Treatment involves local ice application for Grade I reactions. Immediate administration of antivenom is required if any systemic symptoms (Grades II–IV) are identified, especially in children under age 10 years. Any child presenting for a scorpion sting should be admitted to a pediatric intensive care unit. Scorpion stings within residences most frequently occur in the evening due to the scorpion's nocturnal nature and during the summer and early fall months due to high temperatures. Stings occur most often on the extremities. Prevention of stings should be focused on wearing long sleeves and pants if working outside and shaking out clothing and bedding in endemic areas. [36] The public should be aware of the scorpions endemic to the area and the signs and symptoms necessitating presentation to a local medical facility for treatment.

References

1. Blackman JR. Spider bites. J Am Board Fam Pract. 1995;8:288–94.
2. Langley R, Mack K, Haileyesus T, Proescholdbell S, Annest JL. National estimates of non-canine bite and sting injuries treated in US hospital emergency departments, 2001–2010. Wilderness Environ Med. 2014;25(1):14–23.
3. Foelix RF. Biology of spiders. 3rd ed. New York: Oxford University Press; 2011.

4. Wong RC, Hughes SE, Vorhees JJ. Spider bites. Arch Dermatol. 1987;123(1):98–104.
5. Steen CJ, Carbonaro PA, Schwartz RA. Arthropods in dermatology. J Am Acad Dermatol. 2004;50(6):819–42.
6. Isbister GK, White J. Clinical consequences of spider bites: recent advances in our understanding. Toxicon. 2004;43(5):477–92.
7. Diaz JH. The global epidemiology, syndromic classification, management, and prevention of spider bites. Am J Trop Med Hyg. 2004;71(2):239–50.
8. Schwartz RA, Steen CJ. Arthropod bites and stings. In: Goldsmith LA, Katz SI, Gilchrest BA, Paller AS, Leffell DJ, Wolff K, editors. Fitzpatrick's dermatology in general medicine. 8th ed. New York: McGraw-Hill; 2012. Chapter 210.
9. Stoecker WV, Vetter RS, Dyer JA. Not recluse - a mnemonic device to avoid false diagnoses of brown recluse spider bites. JAMA Dermatol. 2017;153(5):377–8.
10. Kang JK, Bhate C, Schwartz RA. Spiders in dermatology. Semin Cutan Med Surg. 2014;33(3):123–7.
11. Diaz JH, Leblanc KE. Common spider bites. Am Fam Physician. 2007;75(6):869–73.
12. Furbee RB, Kao LW, Ibrahim D. Brown recluse spider envenomation. Clin Lab Med. 2006;26(1):211–26.
13. Sams HH, Dunnick CA, Smith ML, King LE. Necrotic arachnidism. J Am Acad Dermatol. 2001;44(4):561–76.
14. Jelinek GA. Widow spider envenomation (latrodectism): a worldwide problem. Wilderness Environ Med. 1997;8(4):226–31.
15. Offerman SR, Daubert GP, Clark RF. The treatment of black widow spider envenomation with antivenin *Latrodectus mactans*: a case series. Perm J. 2011;15(3):76–81.
16. Vetter RS, Isbister GK. Do hobo spider bites cause dermonecrotic injuries? Ann Emerg Med. 2004;44(6):605–7.
17. Vest DK. Protracted reactions following probable hobo spider (*Tegenaria agrestis*) envenomation [abstract]. Am Arachnol. 1993;48:10.
18. Rutzen AR, Weiss JS, Kachodoorian H. Tarantula hair ophthalmia nodosa. Am J Ophthalmol. 1993;116:381–2.
19. Katz TM, Miller JH, Hebert AA. Insect repellents: historical perspective and new developments. J Am Acad Dermatol. 2008;58(5):865–71.
20. Malaque CMS, Vetter RS, Entres M. *Loxosceles* spiders. In: Brent J, Burkhart K, Dargan P, Hatten B, Megarbane B, Palmer R, editors. Critical care toxicology. Cham: Springer; 2015.
21. Gloster HM, Gebauer LE, Mistur RL. Brown recluse spider bite. In: Absolute dermatology review. Cham: Springer; 2016.
22. Vetter RS, Stoecker WV, Dart RC. Envenomations by widow, recluse, and medically implicated spiders. In: Gopalakrishnakone P, Vogel CW, Seifert S, Tambourgi D, editors. Clinical toxicology in Australia, Europe, and Americas. Dordrecht: Springer; 2018. p. 379–412.
23. Pérez-Miles F, Perafán C. Behavior and biology of mygalomorphae. In: Viera C, Gonzaga M, editors. Behaviour and ecology of spiders. Cham: Springer; 2017.
24. Isbister GK, Bawaskar HS. Scorpion envenomation. N Engl J Med. 2014;371(5):457–63.
25. Chippaux JP, Goyffon M. Epidemiology of scorpionism: a global appraisal. Acta Trop. 2008;107(2):71–9.
26. Kang AM, Brooks DE. Nationwide scorpion exposures reported to us poison control centers from 2005 to 2015. J Med Toxicol. 2017;13(2):158–65.
27. Haddad V, Jr., Cardoso JL, Lupi O, Tyring SK. Tropical dermatology: venomous arthropods and human skin: Part II. Diplopoda, Chilopoda, and Arachnida. J Am Acad Dermatol. 2012;67(3):347 e1–9; quiz 55.
28. Pucca MB, Cerni FA, Pinheiro Junior EL, Bordon Kde C, Amorim FG, Cordeiro FA, et al. Tityus serrulatus venom–A lethal cocktail. Toxicon. 2015;108:272–84.
29. Carlson BE, McGinley S, Rowe MP. Meek males and fighting females: sexually-dimorphic antipredator behavior and locomotor performance is explained by morphology in bark scorpions (*Centruroides vittatus*). PLoS ONE. 2014;9(5):e97648.

30. More D, Nugent J, Hagan L, Demain J, Schwertner H, Whisman B, et al. Identification of allergens in the venom of the common striped scorpion. Ann Allergy Asthma Immunol. 2004;93(5):493–8.
31. Khattabi A, Soulaymani-Bencheikh R, Achour S, Salmi LR, Scorpion Consensus Expert G. Classification of clinical consequences of scorpion stings: consensus development. Trans R Soc Trop Med Hyg. 2011;105(7):364–9.
32. LoVecchio F, McBride C. Scorpion envenomations in young children in central Arizona. J Toxicol Clin Toxicol. 2003;41(7):937–40.
33. Boyer LV, Theodorou AA, Berg RA, Mallie J, Arizona Envenomation I, Chavez-Mendez A, et al. Antivenom for critically ill children with neurotoxicity from scorpion stings. N Engl J Med. 2009;360(20):2090–8.
34. Boyer L, Degan J, Ruha AM, Mallie J, Mangin E, Alagon A. Safety of intravenous equine F(ab')2: insights following clinical trials involving 1534 recipients of scorpion antivenom. Toxicon. 2013;76:386–93.
35. Hurst NB, Lipe DN, Karpen SR, Patanwala AE, Taylor AM, Boesen KJ, et al. Centruroides sculpturatus envenomation in three adult patients requiring treatment with antivenom. Clin Toxicol (Phila). 2018;56(4):294–6.
36. Bennett BK, Boesen KJ, Welch SA, Kang AM. Study of factors contributing to scorpion envenomation in arizona. J Med Toxicol. 2019;15(1):30–5.

Arachnida Class: Mites

**David B. Duff, Andrew S. Desrosiers, Robert T. Brodell
and Stephen E. Helms**

Introduction

Mites, along with ticks, make up the subclass Acari within the class Arachnida. These creatures differ from other arachnids in that their bodies are not segmented into cephalothorax and abdomen [1]. While some mites live independently and feed on organic matter, others must parasitize humans and animals in order to sustain life [1]. In this chapter, parasitic mites encountered as outdoor hazards are reviewed with a focus on the clinically significant mites: chiggers and *Cheyletiella*. A few mites less frequently encountered by humans are mentioned in Table 1. Although the scabies mite is a common human affliction, it is not covered in this chapter because it is transmitted via direct human-to-human contact, and is not an outdoor hazard.

D. B. Duff (✉) · A. S. Desrosiers
University of Mississippi School of Medicine, Jackson, MS, USA
e-mail: dduff@umc.edu

A. S. Desrosiers
e-mail: adesrosiers@umc.edu

R. T. Brodell
Professor and Chair, Department of Dermatology, University of Mississippi
School of Medicine, Jackson, MS, USA
e-mail: rbrodell@umc.edu

Professor, Department of Pathology, University of Mississippi
School of Medicine, Jackson, MS, USA

S. E. Helms
Professor of Dermatology, University of Mississippi Medical Center, Jackson, MS, USA
e-mail: sehglh@gmail.com

© Springer Nature Switzerland AG 2020
J. Trevino and A. Y-Y. Chen (eds.), *Dermatological Manual of Outdoor Hazards*,
https://doi.org/10.1007/978-3-030-37782-3_7

Table 1 Mites of Lesser Clinical Significance

Mite:	Common name(s):	Host(s):	Clinical disease(s):	Notes:
	Bird Mites:			
Dermanyssus gallinae (Fig. 1)	Chicken Mite, Red Poultry Mite, Pigeon Mite	Poultry and Wild Birds (Pigeons, Swallows, Starlings, Mynah Birds etc.)	-Avian Mite Dermatitis -Asthma Exacerbation (Inhaled mite or mite feces) [2, 6, 9, 27]	Typically affects agricultural workers who handle infested poultry, but it can also occur as mites enter homes after their bird host nests on windowsills, balconies, rooftops, and attics.
Ornithonyssus bursa	Tropical Fowl Mite			Causes a generalized dermatitis with
Ornithonyssus sylviarum (Fig. 2)	Northern Fowl Mite			widespread pruritic papules that usually affects areas covered by clothing and typically spares the axilla and the genitalia [2, 6, 9, 27]
Ophionyssus bacoti	Tropical Rat Mite	Wild Brown Rat, Black Rat, and other rodents (mice, hamsters, gerbils)	Rat Mite Dermatitis	Causes pruritic, often excoriated papules and wheals Commonly affects areas covered by clothing such as the back, extremities, and wasteline with sparing of the axilla and the genitalia [2, 9]
Ophionyssus natricis (Fig. 3)	Snake Mite	Snakes and Lizards	Snake Mite Dermatitis	Causes pruritic papular and vesicular eruptions in individuals who handle reptiles in their occupation or as pets [2, 9]
Pyemotes spp. (Fig. 4)	Straw Itch Mite, Hay Itch Mite, Grain Itch Mite	Insects found on wheat and other grain-producing plants	Straw Itch (Hay Itch, Grain Itch)	Typically affects workers with occupational exposure to wheat and other grains. Causes intensely pruritic, often excoriated papules with overlying vesicles and may be accompanied by fever, headache, vomiting, and lymphadenopathy [2, 9]

Fig. 1 *Dermanyssus gallinae*: This mite is whitish-gray with four pairs of long legs protruding from an ovoid idiosoma (large posterior portion of the mite which bears the legs). After feeding the body may become engorged and reddish-brown in color Photograph by Alan R Walker—Own work, CC BY-SA 3.0, https://commons.wikimedia.org/w/index.php?curid=19032476

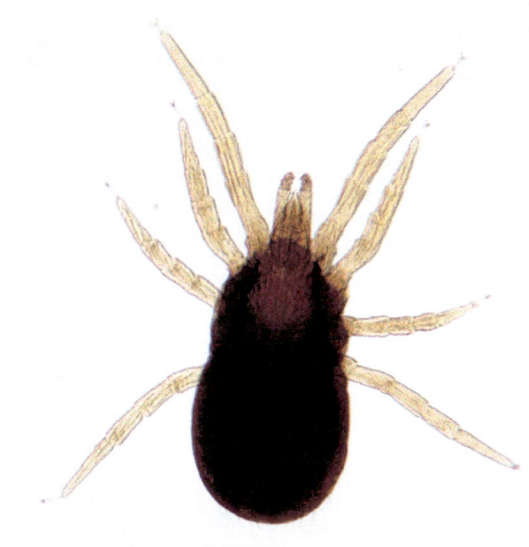

Fig. 2 *Ornithonyssus sylviarum*: This mite closely resembles *Dermanyssus gallinae* with its similar ovoid idiosoma and four pairs of long legs Photograph by Daktaridudu—Own work, CC BY-SA 3.0, https://commons.wikimedia.org/w/index.php?curid=30934182

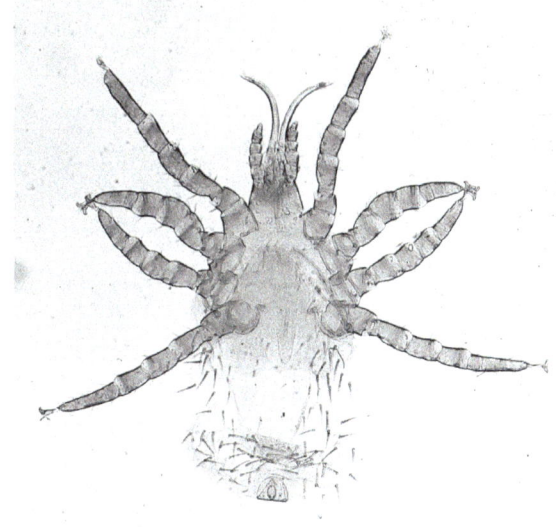

Fig. 3 *Ophionyssus natricis*: This yellow-brown mite has a short, ovoid-to-round idiosoma and may turn dark red or black after feeding. Its first and fourth pairs of legs are longer than the two central pairs Photograph by Dack9—Own work, CC BY 4.0, https://commons. wikimedia.org/w/index. php?curid=73207012

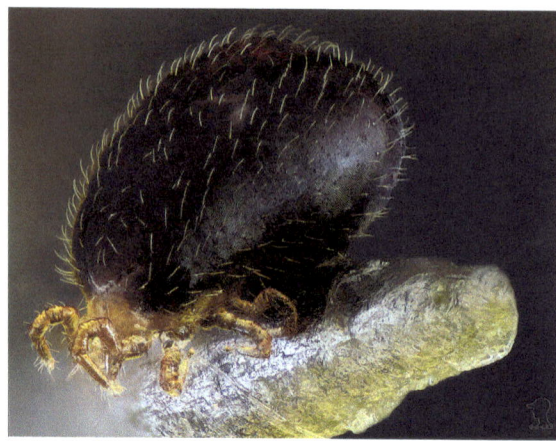

Fig. 4 *Pyemotes* sp.: This mite has a prolate spheroid (football-shaped) idiosoma with two anterior and two posterior leg pairs Photograph by Pavel Klimov, Bee Mite ID (idtools.org/id/mites/ beemites) unless otherwise stated in description on Bee mites website. http://idtools. org/uploads/idtools/37/223/5- BMOC_97-1010-002_ Pyemotes_male_dors_BF100. jpg, CC0, https://commons. wikimedia.org/w/index. php?curid=58419553

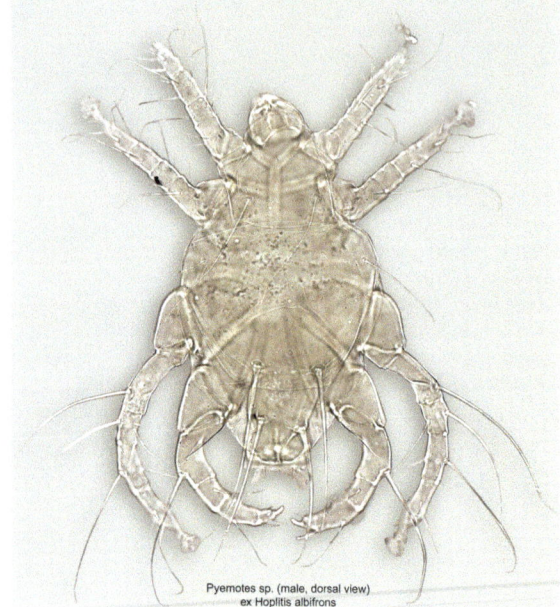

Chiggers

Introduction

Members of the Trombiculidae family of mites, chiggers are also known as harvest mites, harvest bugs, harvest lice, mower's mites, and red bugs [2]. The term "chigger" specifically refers to the 6-legged larval stage of the mite's life cycle and should not be confused with "jigger", a term used to describe the chigoe flea, *Tunga penetrans* [3]. It is only during the larval stage that the mite has the ability to bite its host.

The nymph and adult stages consume vegetation [4]. Chigger bites most frequently occur during summer and early autumn. It is during these seasons that the mites breed and reproduce in large numbers, especially when it is warm and humid and where there is an abundance of grasses, weeds, and other low-lying vegetation [5].

Life Cycle

The life cycle of Trombiculid mites consists of 40 days as they progress through the egg, larval, nymphal, and adult stages. While the mites only complete one annual generation of chiggers in temperate climates (i.e. in summer or early autumn), multiple generations per year can occur in the tropics [6]. Gravid females lay eggs in the soil or on low leaves or grasses, as they require air humidity to be greater than 80% [7]. After a 6 day dormancy period, the eggs hatch into six-legged red chigger larvae [4]. As they wait for a suitable host, the mites remain attached to vegetation less than 30 cm above the ground [7]. While their preferred hosts are small mammals, reptiles and birds, they also infest humans. Larvae feed for up to 1–4 days on their hosts and subsequently detach to continue maturation into the 8-legged nymphal and adult stages [8].

Epidemiology

While Trombiculid mites are found worldwide, habitats are limited to areas in which suitable hosts and moist, grassy environments both exist and are in close proximity to water [4, 9]. *Eutrombicula alfreddugesi* is the predominant species in the southeastern and south central regions of the United States, while *Neotrombicula autumnalis* is more common in Europe and East Asia [2].

Pathogenesis

Chiggers attach to vegetation and wait for a suitable host. Once the chigger transfers to its host, the larvae can travel across the skin for several days [4]. This travel is a deliberate effort to identify the optimal location to latch and begin feeding. Ideal locations are characterized by a thin epidermis and increased air humidity [10, 11]. Consequently, bites are common behind the knees, around the ankles, and between the toes. Waistbands and other areas of tight-fitting clothing serve as barriers to the chigger's exploration, often resulting in clusters of bites around these sites [2]. Once it finds a preferred location, the mites pierce and attach to the host's skin using jaw-like structures called chelicerae [12]. They then form a tube-like opening through the skin called a stylostome by injecting digestive enzymes that liquefy epidermal cells. The stylostome is then used to ingest lymphatic fluid and broken-down tissue [13, 14]. Following the feeding process, the digestive enzymes injected by the mite trigger an immune response that contribute to the characteristic intense pruritus associated with chigger bites [5]. Enzyme-induced cellular mechanical damage and sometimes a superimposed bacterial infection, further contribute to irritation of the skin [4].

Clinical Presentation

While the bites themselves are painless and typically go unnoticed, chigger bites cause cutaneous irritation and inflammation, along with intense pruritus [12, 15]. Post-bite itching is generally delayed by a few hours and typically diminishes within 72 hours. Pruritus, however, may be intense and, on rare occasion, persists for weeks. Bites are characterized as grouped papules or papulovesicles and take 1–2 weeks to completely subside [15]. Bullous, morbilliform, or urticarial eruptions can also occur (Fig. 5) [2, 12].

Diagnosis

No specific tests exist for the confirmation of chigger bites. The classic clinical findings described above combined with a recent history of outdoor activity (especially during the summer and fall) is generally sufficient for diagnosis. On rare occasion and if needed, the diagnosis can be confirmed by retrieving a mite from an infested patient via tape stripping and visualizing the mite with light microscopy [3]. The differential diagnosis for chigger bites may include allergic contact dermatitis, chronic urticaria, other insect bites, scabies, and even urticarial or bullous pemphigoid [3, 5].

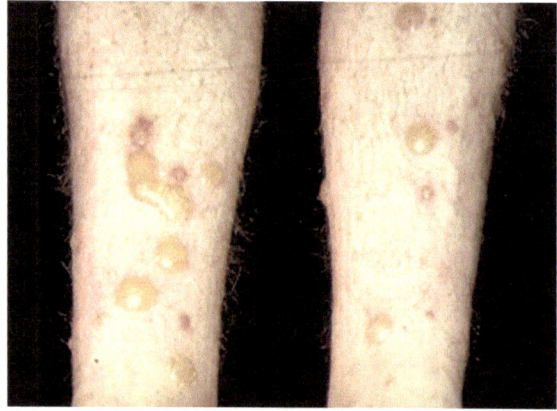

Fig. 5 This patient developed large bullae over the legs following chigger bites

Treatment

Because chiggers detach from the skin soon after feeding and the bites themselves are self-limited, treatment is focused on symptomatic relief. If itching has recently begun, the patient can attempt to remove any remaining larvae by vigorously scrubbing the skin with soap and water. Itching can be managed by topical anti-pruritic agents (e.g., calamine lotion, menthol, pramoxine) or oral antihistamines (e.g., diphenhydramine, hydroxyzine) [4]. Potent topical steroids followed by an occluding plastic wrap may also help alleviate itching and inflammation. Severe pruritus may require intralesional corticosteroids (e.g. 2.5–5 mg/mL of triamcinolone acetonide) or short courses of systemic steroids [9].

Prevention

Precautionary measures should be taken to prevent chigger bites when traveling in infested areas during seasons when larvae are present. The best prevention practices include covering the skin with clothing, tucking shirts into pants and tucking pants into socks. DEET (N,N-diethyl-meta-toluamide) and permethrin can also be applied to clothing and skin [4].

Disease Transmission

Scrub typhus or "tsutsugamushi fever" is a zoonosis of rural areas of Asia and the western Pacific islands. It can be caused by chigger bites in which mites transfer the organism *Orientia tsutsugamushi* to a host via their saliva [16]. Fever, severe headache, and diffuse myalgia are seen, along with an eschar at the site of infection [4]. Treatment with doxycycline 100 mg twice daily is effective [17].

Cheyletiella

Introduction

Cheyletiella are non-burrowing, tiny mites that are nearly invisible to the naked eye (Fig. 6). *Cheyletiella* dermatitis occurs as a result of human contact with an animal infested with the mite, most commonly a pet cat, dog or rabbit. Even animals that are heavily infested with the mite are often asymptomatic, earning it the colloquial name of "walking dandruff." In contrast, humans in contact with these asymptomatic animals experience marked pruritus as the mite feeds on their skin.

Fig. 6 *Cheyletiella*: Both patient and pet rabbit presented to the veterinarian clinic with lesions consistent with insect bites. This mite was found on the body of the rabbit and identified as a cheyletiella mite with its characteristic hooked mouthparts Photograph courtesy of James L. Triggs III, DVM

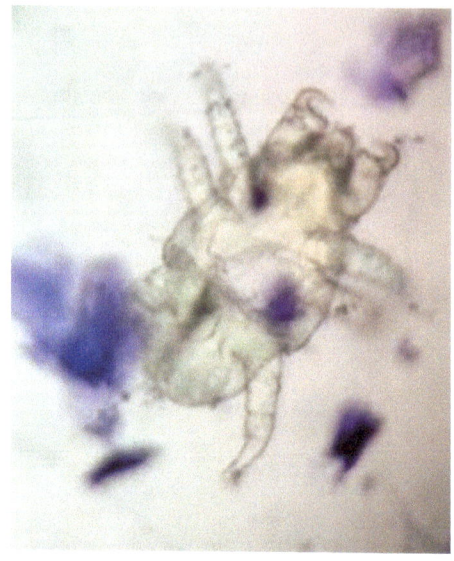

Cutaneous eruptions range from a mild papular rash to a severe reaction causing formation of papules and vesicles that can develop into pustules and become necrotic [18]. *Cheyletiella* mites have a worldwide distribution and are more common in areas where people are in more frequent contact with cats, dogs, or rabbits [19]. It has been estimated that approximately 50% of rabbits in commercial colonies carry *Cheyletiella* [20].

Life Cycle and Pathogenesis

Cheyletiellosis occurs in humans as a result of contact with an infested animal. *Cheyletiella blakei*, *Cheyletiella parasitovorax*, and *Cheyletiella yasguri* affect cats, rabbits, and dogs, respectively [2]. These obligate parasites live in the keratin layer of the host epidermis, where they feed on tissue fluids and surface debris [21]. At approximately 0.4 mm in length, they are difficult to see with the naked eye, appearing as small white specks resembling dandruff on the hair or skin of the host [9]. As many as 20% of pet owners whose pets are infested with *Cheyletiella* become infested themselves [22]. Their life cycle consists of a 35-day period spent on a single host animal, maturing from egg to adult during the first three weeks. While female mites can live up to 10 days after separation from their hosts and can lay eggs during this time, larval, nymph, and adult male mites can only survive for 48 hours apart from their hosts [19].

Clinical Presentation

Infested dogs, cats, and rabbits may be asymptomatic or develop white, scaly patches on the dorsum of the back [23]. In humans, Cheyletiellosis most commonly presents in a female 40 years old or younger with grouped, erythematous, pruritic papules on exposed areas [24]. Grouped vesicles tend to form around areas in direct contact with the infested pet, most commonly the chest, abdomen, and upper extremities (Fig. 7) [25]. Widespread papules, vesicles, bullae, and urticarial wheals occur less frequently [23, 25]. Systemic hypersensitivity to *Cheyletiella blakei* with arthralgia and peripheral eosinophilia has been reported [26].

Diagnosis

Diagnosis can be challenging and requires a high degree of suspicion and knowledge of a patient's animal exposure history [19]. The introduction of a pet into the patient's home environment is a common reason [9]. Generally, a veterinarian must examine the source animal to confirm the presence of *Cheyletiella*. The mite can be identified via brushings, scrapings, or acetate tape preparations from the affected animal [23].

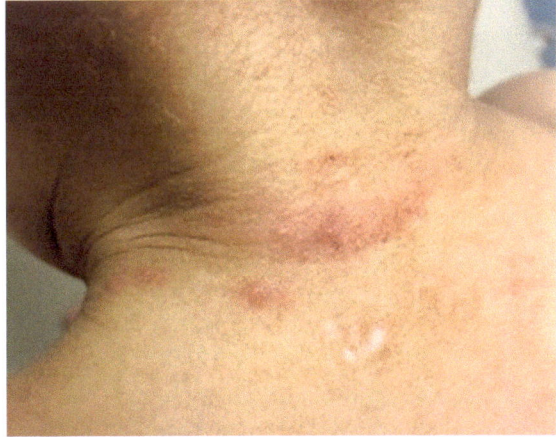

Fig. 7 This patient demonstrated the typical erythematous, pruritic papules in an area of direct contact with a pet infested with *Cheyletiella* mites

Treatment

Cheyletiella infestations are self-limited in humans. Symptoms can be treated with antipruritic medications and topical steroids. Preventing recurrence in the patient relies on identification and treatment of the animal host. Lesions disappear after approximately 3 weeks, provided that the source animal has been treated [19].

Disclosures   None of the authors have relevant conflicts of interest.

References

1. Halliday RB, O'Connor BM, Baker AS. Global diversity of mites. In: Raven PH, Williams T, editors. Nature and human society. Washington, DC: National Academy Press; 1999. p. 192–203.
2. McClain D, Dana AN, Goldenberg G. Mite infestations. Dermatol Ther. 2009;22(4):327–46. https://doi.org/10.1111/j.1529-8019.2009.01245.x.
3. Riemann H, High W. Chigger bites. In: Dellavalle R, Rosen T, Ofori A, editors. UpToDate. Waltham, MA: UpToDate; 2018.
4. Hohenberger ME, Elston DM. What's eating you? chiggers. Cutis. 2017;99(6):386–388. http://www.ncbi.nlm.nih.gov/pubmed/28686755. Accessed 29 Jan 2019.
5. Norris R. Chigger bite in adult. In: Goldsmith L, editor. VisualDx. Rochester, NY: VisualDx; 2018.
6. Varma MRG. Ticks and mites (Acari). In: Lane RP, Crosskey RW, editors. Medical insects and arachnids. 1st ed. London: Chapman & Hall; 1993. p. 597–658.
7. Gasser R, Wyniger R. Distribution and control of Trombiculidae with special reference to Trombicula autumnalis. Acta Trop. 1955;12(4):308–326. http://www.ncbi.nlm.nih.gov/pubmed/13326577. Accessed 29 Jan 2019.
8. Yates VM. Harvest mites–a present from the Lake District. Clin Exp Dermatol. 1991;16(4):277–278. http://www.ncbi.nlm.nih.gov/pubmed/1794169. Accessed 29 Jan 2019.
9. Ken KM, Shockman SC, Sirichotiratana M, Lent MP, Wilson ML. Dermatoses associated with mites other than Sarcoptes. Semin Cutan Med Surg. 2014;33(3):110–115. http://www.ncbi.nlm.nih.gov/pubmed/25577848. Accessed 29 Jan 2019.
10. Jones BM. The penetration of the host tissue by the harvest mite, Trombicul autumnalis Shaw. Parasitology. 1950;40(3–4):247–260. http://www.ncbi.nlm.nih.gov/pubmed/14785964. Accessed 29 Jan 2019.
11. Farkas J. Concerning the predilected localisation of the manifestations of trombidiosis. Predilected localisation and its relation to the ways of invasion. Dermatol Monatsschr. 1979;165(12):858–861. http://www.ncbi.nlm.nih.gov/pubmed/546666. Accessed 29 Jan 2019.
12. Jones JG. Chiggers. Am Fam Phys. 1987;36(2):149–152. http://www.ncbi.nlm.nih.gov/pubmed/3618452. Accessed 29 Jan 2019.
13. Hase T, Roberts LW, Hildebrandt PK, Cavanaugh DC. Stylostome formation by Leptotrombidium mites (Acari: Trombiculidae). J Parasitol. 1978;64(4):712–718. http://www.ncbi.nlm.nih.gov/pubmed/98623. Accessed 29 Jan 2019.
14. Shatrov AB. Stylostome formation in trombiculid mites (Acariformes: Trombiculidae). Exp Appl Acarol. 2009;49(4):261–80. https://doi.org/10.1007/s10493-009-9264-0.

15. Potts J. Eradication of ectoparasites in children. How to treat infestations of lice, scabies, and chiggers. Postgrad Med. 2001;110(1):57–59, 63–64. https://doi.org/10.3810/pgm.2001.07.972.

16. Watt G, Parola P. Scrub typhus and tropical rickettsioses. Curr Opin Infect Dis. 2003;16(5):429–36. https://doi.org/10.1097/01.qco.0000092814.64370.70.

17. Liu Q, Panpanich R. Antibiotics for treating scrub typhus. Cochrane Database Syst Rev. 2002;(2):CD002150. https://doi.org/10.1002/14651858.cd002150.

18. Steen CJ, Carbonaro PA, Schwartz RA. Arthropods in dermatology. J Am Acad Dermatol. 2004;50(6):819–42. https://doi.org/10.1016/j.jaad.2003.12.019.

19. Reynolds HH, Elston DM. What's eating you? Cheyletiella mites. Cutis. 2017;99(5):335,336,355.

20. Flatt RE, Wiemers J. A survey of fur mites in domestic rabbits. Lab Anim Sci. 1976;26(5):758–61.

21. Angarano DW, Parish LC. Comparative dermatology: parasitic disorders. Clin Dermatol. 12(4):543–550.

22. Scott D, Miller W, Griffin C. Parasitic skin diseases. In: Sanders W, editors. Small animal dermatology. 5th ed. Philadelphia; 1995. pp. 412–417.

23. Wagner R, Stallmeister N. Cheyletiella dermatitis in humans, dogs and cats. Br J Dermatol. 2000;143(5):1110–2.

24. Lee BW. Cheyletiella dermatitis: a report of fourteen cases. Cutis. 1991;47(2):111–4.

25. Cvancara JL, Elston DM. Bullous eruption in a patient with systemic lupus erythematosus: mite dermatitis caused by Cheyletiella blakei. J Am Acad Dermatol. 1997;37(2 Pt 1):265–7.

26. Dobrosavljevic DD, Popovic ND, Radovanovic SS. Systemic manifestations of Cheyletiella infestation in man. Int J Dermatol. 2007;46(4):397–9. https://doi.org/10.1111/j.1365-4632.2007.03098.x.

27. Service MW. Miscellaneous Mites. In: Service MW, editor. Medical entomology for students. 1st ed. London: Chapman & Hall; 1996. p. 264–6.

Arachnida Class: Ticks

Maia K. Erickson and Elizabeth M. Damstetter

Introduction

The incidence of tick-borne illnesses in the United States has been increasing dramatically. It is thought that these numbers are vastly underreported due to failures in seeking treatment, misdiagnosis, and lapses in disease reporting. Moreover, not every tick is a carrier of disease nor does every bite by an infected tick transmit disease, so the prevalence of tick bites is difficult to accurately obtain [1]. In practice, some patients may present with the tick still attached, so it is important to be able to identify ticks in order to properly educate and manage patients [2]. When patients present without an attached tick, the bite site initially appears similar to other arthropod bites with a small, erythematous macule, papule, or vesicle that is often intensely pruritic [3].

There are approximately 850 species of ticks known throughout the world, but only 10% are medically relevant. Ticks are generally classified in the families *Ixodidae* (hard ticks), *Argasidae* (soft ticks), and their common ancestor, *Nuttalliellidae* [3]. Hard ticks are responsible for the vast majority of tick-borne illness in humans. They have a hard dorsal plate called a scutum, while soft ticks do not. The differing scutum colors, patterns, and presence of festoons and grooves aid significantly in the correct identification of tick species. Distinguishing features of the most clinically relevant tick genera in the USA are summarized in Table 1 at the end of Sect. "Tick Classification".

All ticks have a similar 4-stage lifecycle which can take up to 3 years to complete. For hard ticks, each stage is associated with a single new host, while soft

M. K. Erickson · E. M. Damstetter (✉)
Department of Dermatology, Rush University Medical Center,
1411 South Michigan Avenue, Chicago, IL 60605, USA
e-mail: liz.damstetter@gmail.com

© Springer Nature Switzerland AG 2020
J. Trevino and A. Y-Y. Chen (eds.), *Dermatological Manual of Outdoor Hazards*,
https://doi.org/10.1007/978-3-030-37782-3_8

ticks tend to live in association with one host throughout all stages. Ticks need blood meals to survive; most ticks die because they cannot find a new host for the next feed [4]. Their lifecycle begins as eggs that hatch into 6-legged larvae, which feed on small woodland mammals or birds. Larvae molt into 8-legged nymphs, which are sexually immature forms of the 8-legged adults; both nymphs and adults feed on large mammals. While some species of larvae and all species of adults may bite and transmit disease to humans, nymphs are the most commonly implicated given their summer feeding activity and their less noticeable, small size [5].

Ticks find their hosts by a variety of mechanisms: some detect body odors or carbon dioxide; others detect heat, moisture, vibrations, or shadows. Employing these sensory measures, they are able to identify well-used host paths and wait on the tips of plants in a process called *questing*, in which the third and fourth pair of legs grasp the plant, and the first pair of legs is outstretched, waiting for a host to brush against it. Some species of tick will attach at the point of contact; others prefer certain locations on the body and will move around before attaching [4].

Ticks are most active from March through October, though this varies by climate. As a result, tick-borne illnesses may present at any time of year [6, 7]. In order to transmit disease, a tick first needs to take a blood meal from an infected host. The pathogen remains in the salivary glands as the tick matures and is then introduced into a new host's dermis from the saliva of the next bite [5]. The risk of transmission of blood-borne diseases increases the longer the tick remains attached. The exact duration of attachment necessary for transmission depends on the pathogen, but prompt removal of ticks significantly reduces the risk of any tick-borne illness. The most medically important ticks in the United States include *Amyblyomma*, *Ixodes*, *Dermacentor*, and *Rhipicephalus*.

Tick Classification

1. *Amblyomma americanum:* "Lone Star Tick" and *Amblyomma maculatum:* "Gulf Coast Tick"

Amblyomma americanum is the most common tick found on humans. This tick lives in the southern United States, ranging from Texas north to Iowa and east to Connecticut [8]. *Amblyomma americanum* can be distinguished by a single white dorsal spot on the female, earning the nickname "Lone Star" tick (Fig. 1). These ticks also have festoons, prominent eyes and long mouth parts. They favor attachment on the legs, buttocks, and groin of their hosts. They are the vectors for many diseases, including human monocytic erlichiosis (HME), Southern tick-associated rash illness (STARI; also known as Missouri Lyme Disease), Heartland virus, Rocky Mountain spotted fever (RMSF), tularemia, American tick bite fever, and

Fig. 1 *Amblyomma americanum* [11]

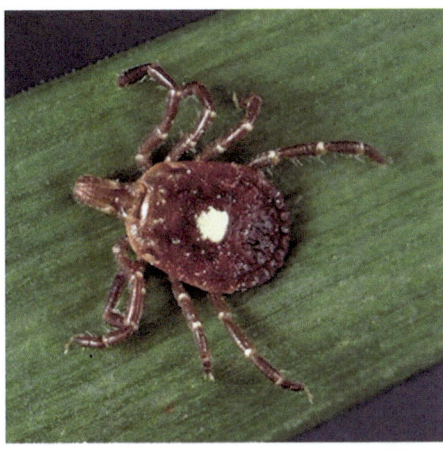

Fig. 2 *Amblyomma maculatum* [12]

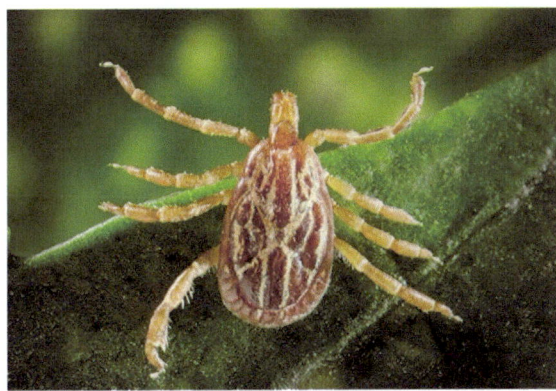

African tick bite fever. They have been implicated in the recently-described alpha-gal syndrome as well [9]. *Amblyomma maculatum* lacks the characteristic white dorsal spot, and instead has a light patterned scutum (Fig. 2). It is found through-out the Atlantic coast and Gulf of Mexico and transmits *Rickettsia parkeri*, which causes a form of spotted fever [10].

2. *Ixodes scapularis*: "Deer Tick", Ixodes *cookei*: "Groundhog tick", and *Ixodes pacificus*: "Western blacklegged tick"

Ixodes scapularis can be identified by its overall teardrop shape with a small plain brown scutum and large underlying cream colored abdomen (Fig. 3). It lacks fes-toons, and has dark legs and short anterior mouthparts. It is most common in the northeastern United States and the Great Lake states, but may be found anywhere

Fig. 3 *Ixodes scapularis* [14]

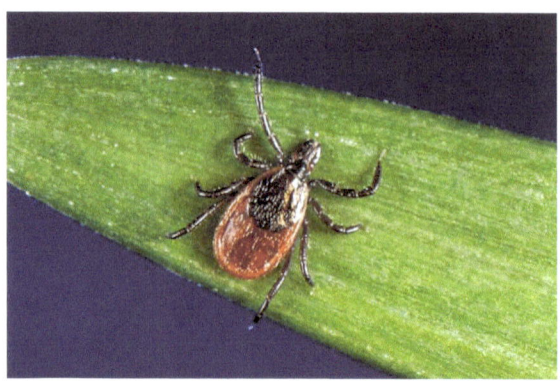

Fig. 4 *Ixodes pacificus* [15]

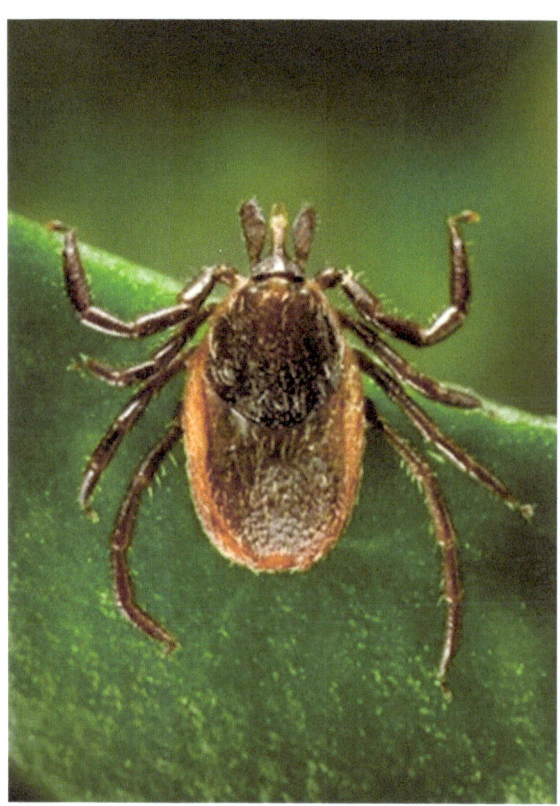

in the eastern United States. These ticks are often found on the trunk. They are an important vector for Lyme disease, human granulocytic anaplasmosis (HGA), and babesiosis [13]. *Ixodes pacificus* (Fig. 4) resides along the Pacific coastal USA and transmits HGA and Lyme disease . *Ixodes cookei* is found in the eastern USA and Canada and transmits a flavivirus causing Powassan disease [10].

3. *Dermacentor andersoni*: "Rocky Mountain Wood Tick" and *Dermacentor variabilis*: "American Dog Tick"

These two species of *Dermacentor* ticks may be distinguished by their geographic locations. As the its nickname implies, *D. andersoni* is confined to the Rocky

Fig. 5 *Dermacentor andersoni* [19]

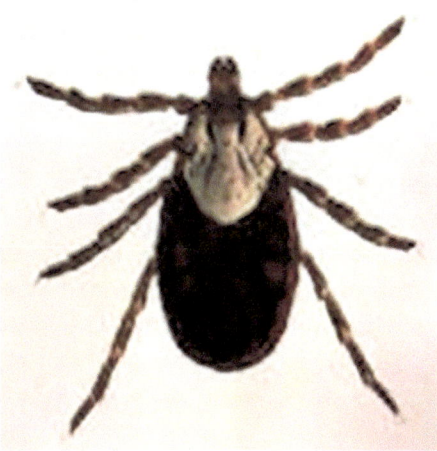

Fig. 6 *Dermacentor variabilis* [20]

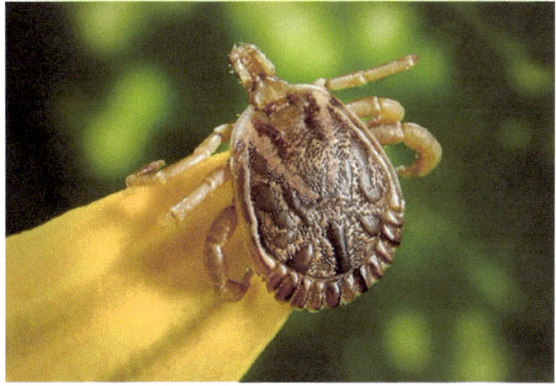

Mountains, whereas *D. variabilis* is distributed throughout the rest of the United States with the exception of the Rocky Mountains. They are less commonly found in heavily wooded areas, and prefer open fields with low vegetation. Both species may be identified by their large, intricate scutum with prominent festoons (Figs. 5 and 6). Their eyes are also prominent, and their mouth parts are small and anterior, erupting from a rectangular basis capituli. Their preferred attachment sites are the head, neck, and shoulder areas. Both species are major vectors for RMSF. They may also transmit tularemia, Q fever, HME, and rickettsial infections [16, 17]. *D. variabilis* is also the vector for Colorado tick fever [18].

4. *Rhipicephalus sanguineus:* **"Brown dog tick"**

Not to be confused with the "American dog tick", *D. variabilis*, *Rhipicephalus sanguineus* may be found indiscriminately throughout the United States and the world. *Rhipicephalus sanguineus* is active all year long, and true to the nickname,

Fig. 7 *Rhipicephalus sanguineus* [24]

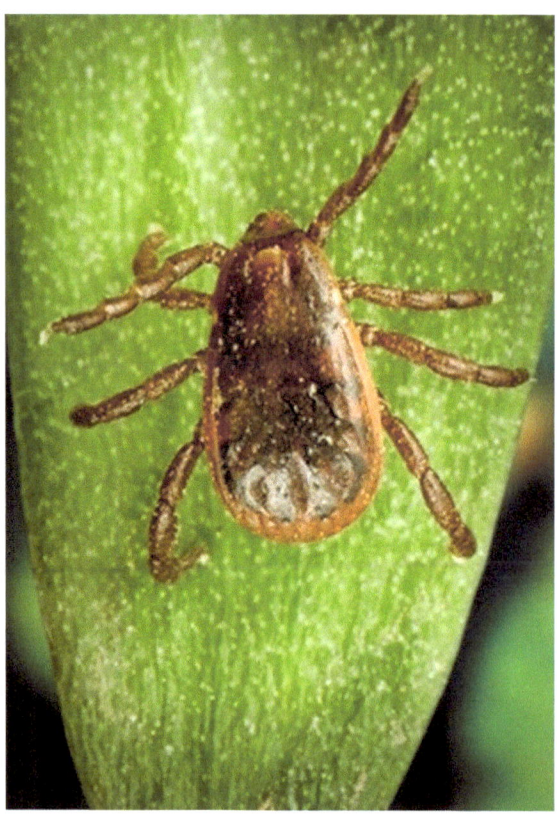

its preferred host species are dogs [21]. In the southwestern United States they most commonly carry RMSF, but they have been known to transmit Boutonneuse fever and Crimean-Congo hemorrhagic fever (CCHF) in other parts of the world [22, 23]. Their appearance is relatively nondescript: a plain, dark brown scutum with deep festoons and prominent eyes (Fig. 7). Their distinguishing feature is a hexagonal basis capituli from which small, anterior mouth parts emerge [16].

5. *Hyalomma*

Hyalomma tick species are not found within the United States. They are more common in Europe, Asia, and Africa, and are most known for carrying CCHF [16]. They may be distinguished by their teardrop shape and banded legs (Fig. 8).

6. *Ornithodoros*

Ornithodoros (Fig. 9) is the one genera of soft tick known to transmit disease to humans, most commonly Borrelial relapsing fever . Different species reside in the west, midwest, and south United States and north Mexico [26]. They are unique in their ability to transmit disease immediately upon attachment.

Fig. 8 *Hyalomma* [25]

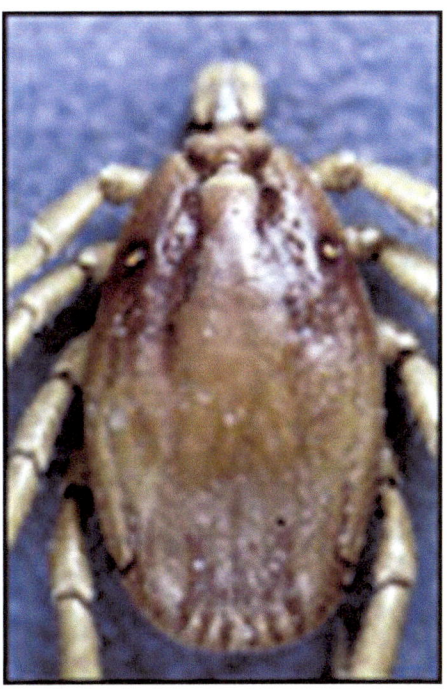

Table 1 Distinguishing features of geographically-relevant tick genera

Tick	Amblyomma	Ixodes	Dermacentor	Rhipicephalus
Appearance	Single white dorsal spot	Dark legs	Ornate scutum	Hexagonal basis capituli
Geographic Distribution	Eastern half of the USA	East Coast and Great Lakes	Isolated to or excluding the Rocky Mountains	Southwest USA
Attachment	Legs, buttocks, groin	Trunk	Head, neck, shoulders	Unspecified
Diseases	RMSF HME Heartland virus American tick bite fever African tick bite fever Tularemia STARI Alpha-gal syndrome	Lyme disease HGA Babesiosis Powassan virus	RMSF HME Colorado tick fever Tularemia Q fever Rickettsial infections	RMSF Boutonneuse Fever CCHF Tularemia

Fig. 9 *Ornithodoros turicata* [27]

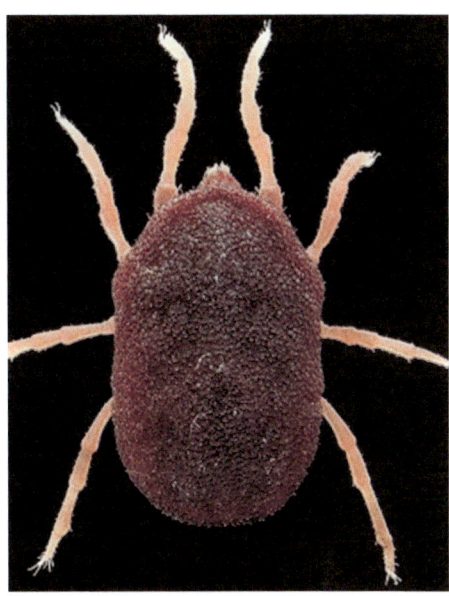

Disease States

1. Lyme Disease

Lyme disease is the most prevalent tick-borne disease in the USA [28]. It is caused by *Borrelia burgdorferi*, a spirochete bacterium found in the northeastern, mid-Atlantic, and north-central USA. This disease is mostly seen in the summer months. Patients with Lyme disease can have concurrent erlichiosis and babesiosis, as all three diseases share common vectors. The species of tick vector depends on the geographic location. The most common vector, *Ixodes scapularis*, is found in the Northeast and Midwest; *Ixodes pacificus* is the vector in the West; *Amblyomma americanum* may transmit *Borrelia* in the South; *Ixodes ricinus* is the main culprit in Europe. The most common reservoir is the white-footed mouse [16].

To transmit *Borrelia*, the tick needs to be attached to its host for more than 48–72 hours [29]. Symptoms onset 3–30 days after the bite. Lyme disease presents in three distinct stages. The hallmark of the early localized phase is *erythema migrans* (EM), an annular erythematous plaque with central clearing or necrosis (Fig. 10). The plaque ranges anywhere from 5 to 70 cm in diameter, and usually involves the legs, groin, or axilla. It is typically asymptomatic itself, but can present with other non-specific constitutional symptoms. EM is the most sensitive indicator of Lyme disease and is present in up to 90% of cases in the United States. It will fade spontaneously in a median time of 28 days [28]. The early disseminated stage occurs 3–5 weeks after the tick bite; the most common presentation is with *multiple* EM, which occurs in 25–50% of patients. Other symptoms seen in early disseminated disease include Bell's palsy, heart block, and peripheral

Fig. 10 Erythema migrans
on the posterior right upper
arm

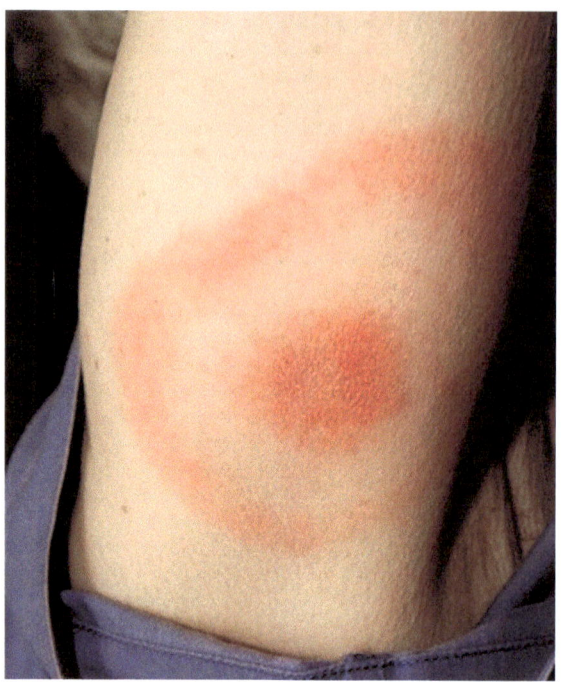

neuropathies. A few months after the initial infection, the late disseminated stage
may occur with a monoarticular arthritis that commonly affects the knee [30].

If at any time Lyme disease is suspected, a screening test for anti-*Borrelia* antibodies such as an ELISA may be employed; however, false positive results may
be seen with conditions such as syphilis, mononucleosis, leptospirosis, or relapsing fever [28, 31]. Therefore, if the screening test is positive, a positive Western
Blot is needed for confirmation. PCR for *B. burgdorferi* DNA is also diagnostic,
but it is less commonly used than the two-test method. Culture is impractical. If
a biopsy is taken from the EM lesion, Warthin-Starry stain reveals spirochetes in
the upper dermis. In practice, the diagnosis is often made clinically simply based
on the presence of EM alone [30]. Of note, an official diagnosis requires clinical
identification of EM in addition to either a proven exposure or laboratory evidence
of infection [16].

Treatment depends on the stage of disease. Doxycycline 100 mg twice a day for
at least 21 days is sufficient for early localized disease. For children 8 years old or
younger and pregnant women, doxycycline is not recommended due to risk of sup-
pression of bone growth and staining of teeth [32]. Instead, amoxicillin for 21 days
is adequate treatment but does not provide the added coverage of *Erlichia*, which
doxycycline does. Pregnant women should receive 500 mg of amoxicillin twice a
day while children are dosed at 20 mg/kg/day. If patients present with Bell's palsy,
first degree heart block, or arthritis, a 28-day course of any of the above listed
regimens may be sufficient. For severe CNS involvement or symptomatic cardiac

arrhythmias, parenteral dosing with penicillin G or a third generation cephalosporin may be employed [30].

Because only 1% of people bitten by ticks develop Lyme disease, routine post-exposure prophylaxis is not recommended. However, if *Ixodes* species can be definitively identified, if the patient was in an endemic area, or if the tick has been attached for >36 hours or is heavily engorged, the risk of infection increases and antibiotic prophylaxis may be indicated. Some providers recommend a single 200 mg dose of doxycycline as prophylaxis; however due to difficult timing, a 10-day oral doxycycline course has more reliable efficacy [16].

2. Human Granulocytic Anaplasmosis

Human granulocytic anaplasmosis (HGA) is caused by *Anaplasma phagocytophilia* groups—obligate intracellular, gram-negative bacteria that have a predilection for neutrophils. This pathogen is found in the northeast and upper midwest USA and is transmitted by the vector *Ixodes scapularis* after 4–24 hours of attachment. Illness presents 1–2 weeks after a tick bite with a nonspecific constitutional symptoms and myalgia. Dermatologic manifestations appear in only 10% of cases, and when present, are also nonspecific. Severity of HGA varies greatly. Because neutrophils are disproportionately targeted, infected patients are at increased risk of opportunistic infections. Hospitalization is required in about one-third of patients, and around 17% of those require ICU support [33]. Around 1% of all patients die from their infection, so treatment with doxycycline 100 mg twice a day for 7 days is recommended if there is a high degree of clinical suspicion. Confirmatory tests include culture, indirect immunofluorescent antibodies, or PCR detection of *Anaplasma phagocytophilia* DNA. Inspection of blood smears may reveal intracytoplasmic inclusion bodies called *morulae* in white blood cells. Doxycycline is the treatment of choice for all patients over the age of 8.

3. Babesiosis

Babesiosis is caused by *Babesia microti*, a parasite that preferentially infects red blood cells. It is found in the northeastern and upper midwestern USA, as well as on other continents. Like Lyme disease, the primary reservoir for babesiosis is the white-footed mouse, and it is transmitted through its vector, *Ixodes scapularis*, after 36–72 hours of attachment. Humans are incidental, terminal hosts. The clinical presentation of babesiosis resembles that of malaria: 1–4 weeks after a tick bite, patients gradually develop malaise, fatigue, myalgia, arthralgia, chills, sweats, anorexia, weight loss, headache, nausea, and a nonproductive cough. Hallmark features include fever and hepatomegaly. Emotional lability, depression, hyperesthesia, photophobia, conjunctival injection, sore throat, abdominal pain, and vomiting may also be seen. Importantly, a rash is not usually present and, if noted, should raise the suspicion for concurrent Lyme disease. Babesiosis can be fatal especially for those whom are older than 50 years of age, immunocompromised, or have had a splenectomy. Diagnosis is made by blood smears with Giemsa stain, detection of *Babesia* DNA by PCR, or by a 4-fold increase in antibody titers. Treatment for mild to moderate disease is atovaquone and azithromycin for 7–10 days. If severe, clindamycin and quinine may be effectively employed. With treatment, symptoms will slowly resolve within 1–2 weeks; however residual fatigue may persist for months [5].

4. Alpha Gal Syndrome

Alpha-gal (galactose-alpha-1, 3 galactose) is an oligosaccharide blood group found in non-primate mammals. Alpha-gal syndrome occurs after an *Amblyomma americanum* tick bite primes an IgE immune response to that oligosaccharide antigen [34, 35]. When alpha-gal is re-encountered through the ingestion of red meat, a delayed anaphylactic or urticarial reaction may occur. This response takes several hours to mount, which often leads to a delay in diagnosis. For unclear reasons, this reaction does not occur every time an affected individual eats red meat. It also seems to occur more frequently if red meat is ingested in association with alcohol, aspirin, or physical activity [36]. The prevalence of this condition is relatively high; one study demonstrated that about one-third of people with significant tick exposure had this immune response primed [37].

Diagnosis is based on the history of red meat exposure 3–5 hours prior to the onset of symptoms in the setting of an individual with prior tick exposure. Alpha-gal IgE titers can be checked, or patients may undergo a skin testing challenge if the initial reaction was mild. Treatment consists of avoidance of red meat. Acute management of an episode involves antihistamines and epinephrine as needed [34].

5. Human Monocytic Erlichiosis

Erlichiosis is caused by *Erlichia chaffeensis*, an obligate intracellular gram-negative bacterium that preferentially infects monocytes. The most common vector is *Amblyomma americanum*, though *Dermacentor variabilis* has been known to transmit erlichiosis as well [38, 39]. This disease most commonly affects 30–60 year-old men in the central, southern, southeastern, and mid-Atlantic United States. It presents 5–21 days after the bite with a nonspecific febrile illness as well as vomiting and diarrhea. Severe forms may involve the kidneys, lungs, and central nervous system. One-third of patients may experience a nonspecific cutaneous eruption on the trunk about 5 days after the fever begins. The cutaneous manifestation is seen more commonly in children. Culture, indirect immunofluorescent antibodies, or PCR are confirmatory tests. Treatment is doxycycline 100 mg twice a day for 7 days for all patients over the age of 8.

6. Rocky Mountain Spotted Fever

Rocky Mountain spotted fever (RMSF) is caused by *Rickettsia rickettsii*, an obligate intracellular gram-negative bacterium. It may be transmitted by multiple vectors, including *Dermacentor andersoni*, *Dermacentor variabilis*, *Rhipicephalus sanguineus*, and *Amblyomma americanum*. The illness presents 1–2 weeks after a

Fig. 11 Characteristic rash of RMSF on the right hand of a child

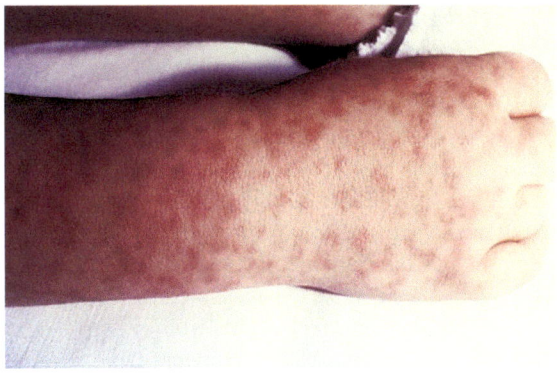

tick bite with an eschar at the bite site, fever, chills, weakness, and hepatomegaly. In 80–90% of cases, blanching, erythematous macules appear on the forehead, palms, soles, wrists, and ankles and spread centrifugally or centripetally over the next 6–18 hours (Fig. 11). The rash becomes petechial and hemorrhagic over the following 2–4 days. Diagnosis is made clinically because antibodies become positive later in the disease course. Mortality of RMSF approaches 60% in older patients. If RMSF is suspected, empiric treatment with doxycycline 100 mg twice a day for 7 days should be started as soon as possible. Treatment must be initiated by the fifth day of illness or mortality increases; it should never be delayed while awaiting confirmatory results [16]. Given its high morbidity and mortality rate, even children younger than 8 years old and pregnant women should receive doxycycline. One-week of doxycycline treatment is unlikely to have adverse effects on dentition or bone growth [32].

7. Tularemia

Tularemia is caused by *Francisella tularensis*, a gram-negative, catalase-positive coccobacillus, an aerobic bacterium. It is transmitted by *Dermacentor andersoni* and *Amblyomma americanum*. The illness presents 3–5 days after the bite with sudden-onset flu-like symptoms. The bite site typically develops a papule that rapidly ulcerates, and regional lymphangitis that leads to suppurative nodules. Erythema multiforme, erythema nodosum, or a macular, papular, vesicular, or petechial exanthem may also be seen [40]. Blood count reveals leukocytosis. Diagnosis is made by culture or fluorescent antibody staining of the exudate. Treatment with intramuscular streptomycin 1 mg every twelve hours for ten days will resolve the illness in six weeks, though scarring may persist.

One important implication of tularemia is the possibility of biowarfare. In addition to being transmitted through arthropod vector bites, it may also be spread through aerosols, contaminated water and food. These routes make intentional dispersion viable, which results in oropharyngeal or pneumonic forms of tularemia [40].

8. Boutonneuse Fever (Mediterranean Spotted Fever)

Boutonneuse fever is caused by *Rickettsia coronii*, an obligate intracellular, gram-negative bacterium transmitted by the vector *Rhipicephalus sanguineus* (Brown dog tick) throughout southern Europe and northern Africa. It most commonly affects children due to their close contact with animals and exposure to the outdoors. The illness begins with a sudden onset high fever, headache, myalgia, abdominal pain, regional lymphadenopathy, and an erythematous maculopapular eruption on the trunk, palms, and soles [41]. A small indurated papule at the bite site, called a *tache noire*, may ulcerate and become necrotic, forming an eschar. Diagnosis is confirmed with serology. Oral doxycycline 100 mg every twelve hours for seven days is the treatment of choice. Azithromycin may be used as a tetracycline alternative in children less than 8 years old. Prognosis is excellent [16].

9. Q Fever

Q fever is a zoonotic disease caused by *Coxiella burnetii*, a universal, gram-negative, obligate intracellular bacterium carried, among others, by arthropod vectors *Rhipicephalus sanguineus*, *Dermacentor andersoni*, and *Amblyomma americanum* [42]. *Coxiella burnetii* is primarily transmitted through aerosolized ruminant feces or birth fluids, and can infect humans and a variety of animals [43, 44]. It presents as a nonspecific febrile illness with an acute or chronic form. In the acute form, the lungs and liver are predominantly affected, resulting in atypical pneumonia and granulomatous hepatitis. Chronic disease affects the heart, leading to culture-negative endocarditis. Dermatologic manifestations are exceedingly rare, but may include erythema nodosum, palatal petechiae, and a vasculitis [44]. Treatment consists of several months of doxycycline; hydroxychloroquine may also be used in some cases.

10. Southern Tick-Associated Rash Illness (STARI)

Southern tick-associated rash illness, or Masters disease, presents very similarly to erythema migrans of Lyme disease, but it is carried by a different tick, *Amblyomma americanum*. The cause of STARI remains unknown. Compared to Lyme disease, STARI is found in a more southern geographic region, occurs earlier in the calendar year, has a shorter incubation period, and boasts a faster recovery time. Patients with STARI were more likely to recall a tick bite and less likely to develop symptoms. The necessity/efficacy of antibiotic treatment is not known [45].

11. Crimean-Congo Hemorrhagic Fever

Worldwide, Crimean-Congo hemorrhagic fever (CCHF) is one of the most common tick-borne illnesses. Commonly affected regions include India, Russia, Eastern Europe, the Middle East, Greece, and Portugal. It is caused by *Nairovirus*, a negative-sense, single-stranded RNA virus and a member of the *Bunyaviridae* family. It is carried by *Hyalomma* species and *Rhipicephalus sanguineus* ticks [23]. The disease is most common in the spring and summer months, and presents

1–3 days after a tick bite with fever, coagulopathy, and hepatitis [46]. Mortality rate approaches 30% [23]. Diagnosis is made by enzyme-linked immunoassay or PCR. The mainstay of treatment is supportive care [46].

12. Colorado Tick Fever

Colorado Tick Fever is caused by *Coltivirus*, a nonenveloped, double-stranded RNA virus with a segmented genome. It is transmitted by *Dermacentor andersoni* throughout the western United States and Canada. Symptoms occur 2–3 days after a tick bite, and consist of a triad of acute onset biphasic fever, headache, and myalgia. The illness lasts for 3 weeks or longer due to the persistent infection of red blood cells, but is typically self-limited. The best diagnostic tests include serology and PCR, which are both more accurate than the previous method of detecting serum IgM. Still, a convalescent-phase serum analysis 2 weeks after illness onset is required for diagnosis. Treatment is supportive care [47].

13. African Tick Bite Fever

African tick bite fever is caused by the bacteria *Rickettsia africae*. It is transmitted through *Amblyomma hebraeuem* in southern Africa and through *Amblyomma variegatum* in all other parts of Africa and the Caribbean Islands. In addition to a nonspecific febrile illness and myalgia, 50% of patients will get a nonspecific rash that presents within 3–5 days of the tick bite. The bite site often becomes erythematous with an eschar with surrounding regional lymphadenopathy [16]. Management consists of doxycycline for 7 days [48].

14. American Tick Bite Fever (Maculatum Disease)

American tick bite fever is caused by *Rickettsia parkeri* and is transmitted through *Amblyomma americanum* and *Amblyomma maculatum* throughout North and South America. In contrast to African tick bite fever, up to 80% of patients develop a nonspecific rash within 2–4 days of a tick bite with mild constitutional symptoms [16]. As with all rickettsial infections, doxycycline is the treatment of choice [49].

15. Tick Paralysis

Tick paralysis is a rare but severe complication of a tick bite that results in bilateral ascending flaccid paralysis. It is caused by a neurotoxin produced by *Dermacentor andersoni*; symptoms occur in the host after a female tick has been feeding on it for 5–7 days [50, 51]. The presentation begins with irritability, fatigue, myalgia, and paresthesia; shortly after, ataxia, areflexia, and ascending paralysis develop. The symptoms peak 24–48 hours after onset [52]. The condition resolves rapidly with removal of the tick, which is both diagnostic and therapeutic [53]. The geographic distribution is concentrated in the northwestern United States, and the vast majority of cases occur between April and June [55].

Prevention of Tick-Borne Illness

The role of prevention in tick-borne illnesses cannot be overstated. The most effective method of prophylaxis is through the prevention of tick attachment. Removing animal hosts or treating them for common pathogens may reduce transmission of disease. Avoiding leafy debris and vegetation, such as long grasses and wooded areas, during peak tick seasons is advisable. Wearing long, tightly secured, protective clothing will also be of benefit. Additionally, permethrin impregnated clothing, shoes, and bed nets offer additional protection against tick bites [56].

Checking for ticks after high-risk environmental exposures is another critical component of prevention. If a tick is identified, it should be promptly and properly removed to prevent disease transmission. Lyme disease and babesiosis, typically require greater than 24 hours of tick attachment for transmission [56]. Tweezers or commercially available tick removal devices should be used to grasp the tick behind the mouth parts without squeezing the abdomen. Traction should be applied until the tick releases its grasp [2]. Twisting is generally not advised as it may result in inadvertently leaving residual mouthparts in the skin.

In general, antibiotic prophylaxis after tick bites is not recommended, although RMSF and Lyme disease are exceptions to this rule. Instead, normal-risk bite sites should be regularly inspected for one month to insure that no signs of disease develop [2]. If the risk of disease transmission is high, prophylactic oral doxycycline may be considered; however, a single dose is difficult to time correctly given the highly variable transmission rates and incubation periods, so a 10-day treatment course of doxycycline is often preferable [16].

Correct identification of the biting tick is of extreme importance in determining potential infectious risks and prescribing management/treatment. In addition to standard resources to assist with identification of recovered ticks, a photo can be submitted to tickencounter.org (site sponsored by the University of Rhode Island) to assist with accurate tick identification.

References

1. Gleim ER, Garrison LE, Vello MS, Savage MY, Lopez G, Berghaus RD, et al. Factors associated with tick bites and pathogen prevalence in ticks parasitizing humans in Georgia, USA. Parasit Vectors. 2016;9:125.
2. Aberer E. What should one do in case of a tick bite? Curr Probl Dermatol. 2009;37:155–66.
3. Haddad V Jr, Haddad MR, Santos M, Cardoso JLC. Skin manifestations of tick bites in humans. An Bras Dermatol. 2018;93(2):251–5.
4. How ticks spread disease Cdc.gov: CDC; 2019. https://www.cdc.gov/ticks/life_cycle_and_hosts.html.
5. Vannier EG, Diuk-Wasser MA, Ben Mamoun C, Krause PJ. Babesiosis. Infect Dis Clin North Am. 2015;29(2):357–70.

6. Brugger K, Walter M, Chitimia-Dobler L, Dobler G, Rubel F. Seasonal cycles of the TBE and Lyme borreliosis vector Ixodes ricinus modelled with time-lagged and interval-averaged predictors. Exp Appl Acarol. 2017;73(3–4):439–50.

7. Hayes LE, Scott JA, Stafford KC 3rd. Influences of weather on Ixodes scapularis nymphal densities at long-term study sites in Connecticut. Ticks Tick Borne Dis. 2015;6(3):258–66.

8. Springer YP, Eisen L, Beati L, James AM, Eisen RJ. Spatial distribution of counties in the continental United States with records of occurrence of Amblyomma americanum (Ixodida: Ixodidae). J Med Entomol. 2014;51(2):342–51.

9. Reynolds HH, Elston DM. What's eating you? lone star tick (Amblyomma americanum). Cutis. 2017;99(2):111–4.

10. Tickborne diseases of the United States: A reference manual for health care providers cdc. gov: CDC; 2017, 4th ed. https://www.cdc.gov/lyme/resources/tickbornediseases.pdf.

11. Gathany JLM. Amblyomma americanum. Wikimedia Commons: Center for Disease Control and Prevention; 2003.

12. Gathany JPC. Amblyomma maculatum. Wikimedia Commons: Center for Disease Prevention and Control; 2008.

13. Nelder MP, Russell CB, Sheehan NJ, Sander B, Moore S, Li Y, et al. Human pathogens associated with the blacklegged tick Ixodes scapularis: a systematic review. Parasit Vectors. 2016;9:265.

14. Gathany JLM. Ixodes scapularis. Wikimedia Commons: Center for Disease Control and Prevention; 2009.

15. Gathany JLA, Nicholson W, Reeves W, Paddock C. Ixodes pacificus. Wikimedia Commons: Center for Disease Control and Prevention; 2005.

16. Bolognia JJ, Schaffer J, editors. Dermatology, 3rd ed. Elsevier Saunders; 2012.

17. Hudman DA, Sargentini NJ. Prevalence of tick-borne pathogens in Northeast Missouri. Mo Med. 2018;115(2):162–8.

18. Klasco R. Colorado tick fever. Med Clin North Am. 2002;86(2):435–40, ix.

19. Dermacentor andersoni. Wikimedia Commons: Center for Disease Control and Prevention; 2009.

20. Pixabay. Brown Tick on Yellow Leaf in Close-up Photography. Pexels.com. p. https://www.pexels.com/photo-license/.

21. Nagamori Y, Payton M, Coburn L, Thomas JE, Reichard M. Nymphal engorgement weight predicts sex of adult Amblyomma americanum, Amblyomma maculatum, Dermacentor andersoni, Dermacentor variabilis, and Rhipicephalus sanguineus ticks. Exp Appl Acarol. 2019;77(3):401–10.

22. Villarreal Z, Stephenson N, Foley J. Possible Northward introgression of a tropical lineage of rhipicephalus sanguineus ticks at a site of emerging Rocky Mountain Spotted Fever. J Parasitol. 2018;104(3):240–5.

23. Sharifinia N, Rafinejad J, Hanafi-Bojd AA, Chinikar S, Piazak N, Baniardalan M, et al. Hard ticks (Ixodidae) and Crimean-Congo hemorrhagic fever virus in south west of Iran. Acta Med Iran. 2015;53(3):177–81.

24. Rhipicephalus sanguineus. Wikimedia Commons; 2006.

25. Hyalomma. Wikimedia Commons: Center for Disease Control and Prevention; 2006.

26. Donaldson TG, Perez de Leon AA, Li AY, Castro-Arellano I, Wozniak E, Boyle WK, et al. Assessment of the geographic distribution of Ornithodoros turicata (Argasidae): climate variation and host diversity. PLoS Negl Trop Dis. 2016;10(2):e0004383.

27. Detail, Tick Species Page Ornithodoros turicata TA-367-0516 (page 2 crop). Wikimedia Commons: U.S. Army Center for Health Promotion and Preventative Medicine; 2016.

28. James W, Elston D, editors. Andrews' diseases of the skin, 11th ed. Saunders Elsevier; 2011.

29. Piesman J, Mather TN, Sinsky RJ, Spielman A. Duration of tick attachment and Borrelia burgdorferi transmission. J Clin Microbiol. 1987;25(3):557–8.

30. Murray TS, Shapiro ED. Lyme disease. Clin Lab Med. 2010;30(1):311–28.
31. Miller JM, Binnicker MJ, Campbell S, Carroll KC, Chapin KC, Gilligan PH, et al. A guide to utilization of the microbiology laboratory for diagnosis of infectious diseases: 2018 update by the Infectious Diseases Society of America and the American Society for Microbiology. Clin Infect Dis. 2018;67(6):813–6.
32. Cross R, Ling C, Day NP, McGready R, Paris DH. Revisiting doxycycline in pregnancy and early childhood–time to rebuild its reputation? Expert Opin Drug Saf. 2016;15(3):367–82.
33. Bakken JS, Dumler JS. Human granulocytic anaplasmosis. Infect Dis Clin North Am. 2015;29(2):341–55.
34. Platts-Mills TA, Schuyler AJ, Tripathi A, Commins SP. Anaphylaxis to the carbohydrate side chain alpha-gal. Immunol Allergy Clin North Am. 2015;35(2):247–60.
35. Araujo RN, Franco PF, Rodrigues H, Santos LCB, McKay CS, Sanhueza CA, et al. Amblyomma sculptum tick saliva: alpha-Gal identification, antibody response and possible association with red meat allergy in Brazil. Int J Parasitol. 2016;46(3):213–20.
36. Ohta T, Yoshikawa S, Tabakawa Y, Yamaji K, Ishiwata K, Shitara H, et al. Skin CD4(+) memory T cells play an essential role in acquired anti-tick immunity through interleukin-3-mediated basophil recruitment to tick-feeding sites. Front Immunol. 2017;8:1348.
37. Fischer J, Lupberger E, Hebsaker J, Blumenstock G, Aichinger E, Yazdi AS, et al. Prevalence of type I sensitization to alpha-gal in forest service employees and hunters. Allergy. 2017;72(10):1540–7.
38. Paddock CD, Childs JE. Ehrlichia chaffeensis: a prototypical emerging pathogen. Clin Microbiol Rev. 2003;16(1):37–64.
39. Schutze GE, Buckingham SC, Marshall GS, Woods CR, Jackson MA, Patterson LE, et al. Human monocytic ehrlichiosis in children. Pediatr Infect Dis J. 2007;26(6):475–9.
40. Carvalho CL, Lopes de Carvalho I, Ze-Ze L, Nuncio MS, Duarte EL. Tularaemia: a challenging zoonosis. Comp Immunol Microbiol Infect Dis. 2014;37(2):85–96.
41. Peixoto S, Ferreira J, Carvalho J, Martins V. Mediterranean spotted fever in children: study of a Portuguese Endemic Region. Acta Med Port. 2018;31(4):196–200.
42. Q-Fever Stop Ticks On People: Families First New York Inc.; 2009. http://www.stopticks. org/ticks/qfever.asp.
43. Duron O, Sidi-Boumedine K, Rousset E, Moutailler S, Jourdain E. The importance of ticks in Q fever transmission: What Has (and Has Not) been demonstrated? Trends Parasitol. 2015;31(11):536–52.
44. Salifu SP, Bukari AA, Frangoulidis D, Wheelhouse N. Current perspectives on the transmission of Q fever: highlighting the need for a systematic molecular approach for a neglected disease in Africa. Acta Trop. 2019;193:99–105.
45. Wormser GP, Masters E, Nowakowski J, McKenna D, Holmgren D, Ma K, et al. Prospective clinical evaluation of patients from Missouri and New York with erythema migrans-like skin lesions. Clin Infect Dis. 2005;41(7):958–65.
46. Ergonul O. Crimean-Congo haemorrhagic fever. Lancet Infect Dis. 2006;6(4):203–14.
47. Brackney MM, Marfin AA, Staples JE, Stallones L, Keefe T, Black WC, et al. Epidemiology of Colorado tick fever in Montana, Utah, and Wyoming, 1995-2003. Vector Borne Zoonotic Dis. 2010;10(4):381–5.
48. Mack I, Ritz N. African Tick-Bite Fever. N Engl J Med. 2019;380(10):960.
49. Other spotted fever rickettsioses: Information for health care providers CDC.gov: CDC; 2019. http://www.cdc.gov/otherspottedfever/healthcare-providers/index.html.
50. Greenstein P. Tick paralysis. Med Clin North Am. 2002;86(2):441–6.
51. Gordon BM, Giza CC. Tick paralysis presenting in an urban environment. Pediatr Neurol. 2004;30(2):122–4.
52. Diaz JH. A comparative meta-analysis of tick paralysis in the United States and Australia. Clin Toxicol (Phila). 2015;53(9):874–83.
53. Laufer CB, Chiota-McCollum N. A case of subacute ataxia in the summertime: tick paralysis. J Gen Intern Med. 2015;30(8):1225–7.

54. Dworkin MS, Shoemaker PC, Anderson DE. Tick paralysis: 33 human cases in Washington State, 1946-1996. Clin Infect Dis. 1999;29(6):1435–9.
55. Morshed M, Li L, Lee MK, Fernando K, Lo T, Wong Q. A retrospective cohort study of tick paralysis in British Columbia. Vector Borne Zoonotic Dis. 2017;17(12):821–4.
56. Miller NJ, Rainone EE, Dyer MC, Gonzalez ML, Mather TN. Tick bite protection with permethrin-treated summer-weight clothing. J Med Entomol. 2011;48(2):327–33.

Insecta Beetles, Bees, Wasps, Ants

Gloria Lin, Madeline DeWane and Diane Whitaker-Worth

Beetles

Beetles (order Coleoptera) comprise the largest order of the insect class with over 350,000 species. They exhibit tremendous variability with respect to ecology, biology, and morphology. Much of their success as an order can be attributed to their defensive mechanisms, including sclerotized body structures that provide protection from a variety of environmental hazards, and caustic substances which can be secreted to deter would-be predators [1]. Multiple families of beetles can cause dermatitis, either through the release of irritant chemicals or via mechanical mechanisms; these include Meloidae (blister beetles), Oedemeridae ("false" blister beetles), Dermestidae (carpet, hide, or larder beetles), and Staphlinidae (rove beetles).

Blister Beetles

Meloidae, also known as "blister beetles," are a family comprised of over 125 genera and 3000 species [2]. These insects are often brightly colored, vary between 10 and 15 mm in length, and have long, slender bodies (Fig. 1) [3]. Lytta vesicatoria (responsible for producing the blistering agent "Spanish fly") is probably the most well-known, but Meloidae are found worldwide and across North America with

G. Lin · M. DeWane · D. Whitaker-Worth (✉)
Dermatology Department, University of Connecticut, 21 South Road, Farmington, CT 06032, USA
e-mail: whitaker@uchc.edu

G. Lin
e-mail: glin@uchc.edu

M. DeWane
e-mail: dewane@uchc.edu

© Springer Nature Switzerland AG 2020
J. Trevino and A. Y-Y. Chen (eds.), *Dermatological Manual of Outdoor Hazards*,
https://doi.org/10.1007/978-3-030-37782-3_9

Fig. 1 Lytta vesicatoria.
**By Siga—Own work, CC
BY-SA 3.0** https://commons.
wikimedia.org/w/index.
php?curid=15982308

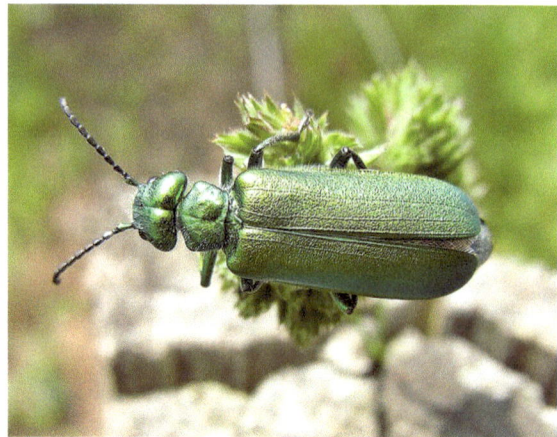

Fig. 2 Intraepidermal blister
resulting from cantharidin
exposure. From Dieterle,
R., Faulde, M. & Erkens,
K. Hautarzt (2015) 66: 370
https://doi.org/10.1007/
s00105-015-3603-3

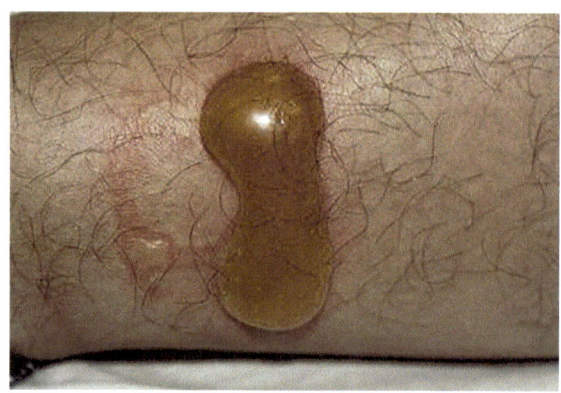

the greatest diversity found in warm, dry climates [4]. Since their diet consists of leaves and crops, they often come into contact with humans, who regard them as agricultural pests [5].

Meloidae are best known for their defensive secretion of cantharidin, a vesicating agent. Cantharidin easily penetrates the epidermis and is absorbed into the lipid component of keratinocyte membranes where it activates serine proteases and degenerates desmosomes [6]. This results in intraepidermal blister formation and acantholysis. A vesiculobullous eruption usually occurs within hours of contact with the beetle (Fig. 2). Treatment is supportive, and lesions typically heal without scarring. Multiple cases of "Meloidae dermatitis" or "blister beetle dermatitis" have been reported in the literature in a variety of geographic locations [7–9].

Although historically cantharidin produced by Meloidae beetles was used as an aphrodisiac [10], it is also of medical interest due to its therapeutic benefits (e.g. a blistering agent in the treatment of verruca vulgaris and molluscum contagiosum) [6].

"False" Blister Beetles

There are approximately 1500 species of Oedemeridae beetles. These beetles also produce cantharidin and are therefore referred to as "false" blister beetles. They have blue, yellow, orange, or red markings and range from 5–20 mm in length. They are found in foliage or around flowers, and feed on pollen [7, 11]. Oedemeridae species are more prevalent in the southern United States, and they are especially common in the Florida Keys [12].

Oedemeridae dermatitis is similar to Meloidae dermatitis as both are caused by exposure to cantharidin, but lesions caused by Oedemeridae species tend to be smaller due to the insects' relatively smaller size [7]. Similar to blister beetle dermatitis, Oedmeridae dermatitis is characterized by a vesiculobullous eruption that occurs hours after beetle contact and is associated with minimal erythema of the surrounding skin. Lesions are typically asymptomatic and most commonly found on the neck, arms, and trunk. Complete healing occurs in 7–10 days [13].

Cases of Oedemeridae dermatitis have been reported worldwide, including the Pacific Islands [14], Bahamas (Genera Alloxacis and Oxacis) [15], Papua New Guinea (Eobia kanack) [16], Puerto Rico (Oxycopis vittata) [17], New Zealand (Thelyphassa lineata) [13], Hawaiian Islands (Thelyphassa apicata) [18], Caribbean (Oxycopis mcdonaldi), and the Florida Keys (Oxycopis mcdonaldi) [12].

Carpet, Hide, or Larder Beetles

The family Dermestidae includes approximately 700 species that are also known as carpet, hide, or larder beetles. Historically, these beetles were considered to be household pests, which live behind baseboards or molding, within heating systems, furniture, or clothing causing damage particularly under heavy furniture and carpet edges. They are excellent scavengers and can feed on a variety of plant and animal substances, including furs, skins, feathers, horns, hair, seeds, grains, dead insects, and bird and rodent nests [19]. They are well known for feeding on carcasses and picking them clean. For example, Dermestidae beetles are used by taxidermists and natural history museums to clean animal specimens [20] and in forensic entomology [21]. Dermestidae beetles are brown or black in color, vary in shape, and range from 1–12 mm in length (Fig. 3) [22]. They are ubiquitous within the United States; Attagenus megatoma and Anthrenus scrophulariae are the most prevalent species [23].

Unlike Meloidae and Oedmeridae, Dermestidae do not produce cantharidin or chemical irritants. Instead, their larvae are covered in hairs (hastae), which break off and are carried by air currents. Hastae (Fig. 4) can penetrate the skin and mucous membranes, causing histamine release and dermatitis . Respiratory problems can occur if the hairs are inhaled [10]. Lymphadenopathy, allergic rhinitis,

Fig. 3 Anthrenus museorum.
By Siga—Own work, Public
Domain https://commons.
wikimedia.org/w/index.
php?curid=2708587

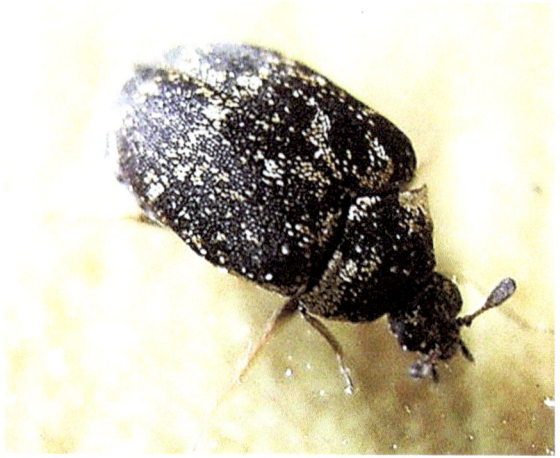

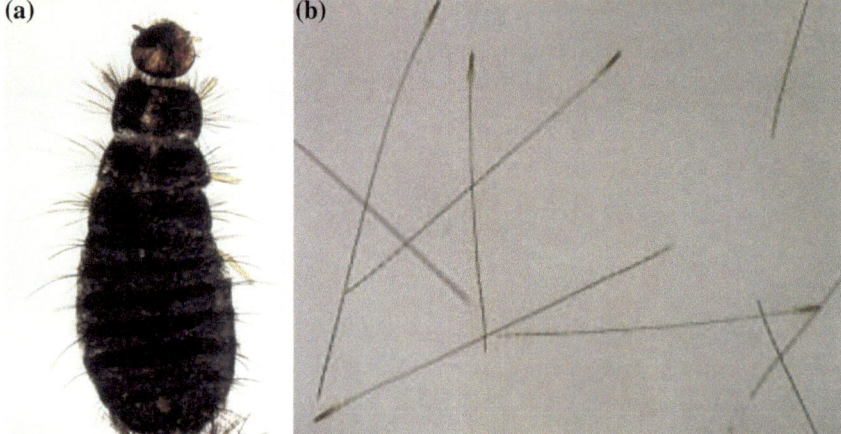

Fig. 4 Dermestid beetle larva (a) and larval hastae under light microscopy (b). From Horster, S.,
Prinz, J., Holm, N. et al. Hautarzt (2002) 53: 328 https://doi.org/10.1007/s001050100257

and vasculitis have also been reported [24]. Cases have been described in Scotland,
North Africa, Austria, Italy, Germany, Britain, and the United States [23, 25–27].

Dermestid dermatitis is characterized by pruritic erythematous urticarial or pap-
ulopustular eruptions. Since the reaction is due to larval hairs and not to the beetle
itself, flares can wax and wane and may persist even after the beetles have been
eradicated [23]. The hypersensitivity component of Dermestid dermatitis is supported by case reports of positive skin or patch testing using both larval extract
(made from dried, ground larvae), as well as with unprocessed, decapitated larvae
or larval hairs applied directly to the skin [23, 25, 28]. Due to its rare nature and
non-specific clinical presentation, there are reports of Dermestid dermatitis being
misdiagnosed as delusions of parasitosis [27].

The treatment of Dermestid dermatitis is primarily symptomatic and includes topical corticosteroids, anti-histamines, and anti-pruritic agents. Definitive treatment is aimed at controlling infestation via fumigation and/or thorough vacuuming [23, 24].

Rove Beetles

The family Staphilinidae, best known for its rove beetles, includes several hundred species distributed throughout Europe, Africa, South America, Asia, and Australia. Staphilinids typically have long slender bodies approximately 5–10 mm in length (Fig. 5) [29].

Easily recognized by the shells (elytra) overlying their wings [5], Staphilinids can fly, but prefer to crawl and have a characteristic habit of curling up when distressed. They tend to be attracted to white lights at night, and they do not bite or sting [29]. Although Staphilinids are most often found living in crops in hot, arid climates, there have been reports of dermatitis caused by Staphilinids in the southwestern United States [8]. With global temperatures increasing, the Staphilinidae family is likely to become more prevalent in the southern US in the future [30].

The dermatitis caused by Staphilinidae beetles is well-characterized and has been described as blister beetle dermatitis, acid beetle dermatitis, night burn, rove beetle dermatitis, whiplash dermatitis, and dermatitis linearis. It is caused by paederin, a crystalline, caustic amide that acts as a vesicant and interferes with mitosis by interacting with cellular DNA [5]. Production of paederin relies on an endosymbiont Pseudomonas species and primarily occurs in adult female beetles [31].

Fig. 5 Dorsal (**a**) and ventral (**b**) views of Paederus fuscipes. From Prasher, P., Kaur, M., Singh, S. et al. Int Ophthalmol (2017) 37: 885 https://doi.org/10.1007/s10792-016-0352-y

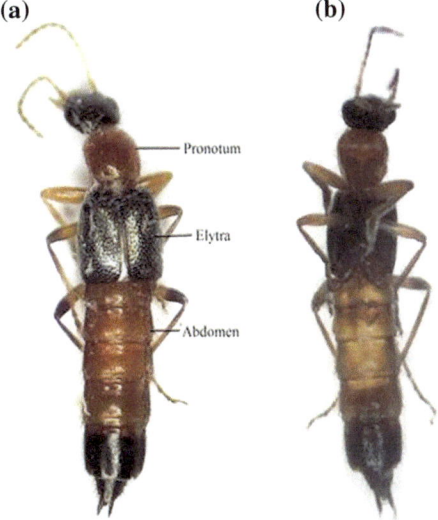

Dermatitis occurs when a beetle is inadvertently crushed thereby exposing the skin to the beetle's hemolymph and coelomic fluid, which contains the paederin [30].

Unlike cantharidin reactions, which are non-inflammatory, paederus dermatitis is characterized by vesicles, bullae, and pustules on intensely inflamed skin that arises within 24 hours of contact with a Staphilinid species (Fig. 6a) [32, 33].

The eruption is often accompanied by a burning or stinging sensation which may be misdiagnosed as herpes simplex or herpes zoster [30]. Other diagnoses with a similar clinical picture include burns, acute allergic contact dermatitis, phytophotodermatitis, bullous impetigo, and dermatitis artefacta [32]. Classical clinical findings include "kissing lesions" (Fig. 6b) from local spread of the irritant between opposing flexural surfaces and linear "whiplash lesions." [33] Outbreaks of Paederus dermatitis have been reported in Malaysia, Sri Lanka, Egypt, Nigeria, Iran, Iraq, Central China, Africa, Guinea, France, Venezuela, Ecuador, Australia, and Turkey, [29, 34–39] as well as a single case report in the United States that involved 33 military personnel in Arizona with consistent symptoms [32].

Once identified, paederus dermatitis should be managed as any other irritant contact dermatitis with prompt washing, cold compresses, and topical corticosteroids [33]. Tincture of iodine may also be helpful as a solvent for early lesions while vesicles, crusts, and pustules can be treated with potassium permanganate. Topical or systemic antibiotics may be required for secondary infections [5]. Lesions typically heal in 10–14 days, and post-inflammatory dyschromia is common [39]. More serious complications have also been reported. Extensive exfoliating or ulcerating dermatitis may require hospitalization [40], and systemic

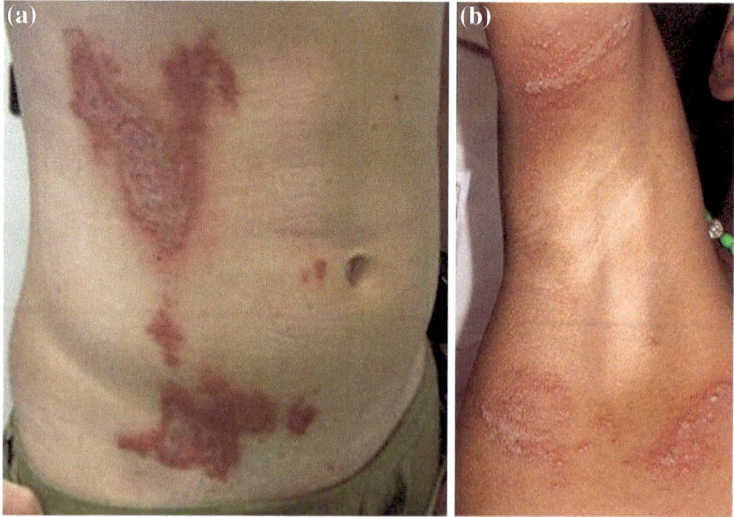

Fig. 6 Paederus dermatitis. Vesicles and pustules on inflamed, erythematous skin (**a**) and a classic "kissing lesion" from paederin spread between opposing skin surfaces (**b**). From Dieterle, R., Faulde, M. & Erkens, K. Hautarzt (2015) 66: 370 https://doi.org/10.1007/s00105-015-3603-3

symptoms including fever, neuralgia, arthralgia, and vomiting may occur when skin involvement is widespread [41]. Genital or ocular involvement, sometimes referred to as "Nairobi eye," [34, 40, 42, 43] may result when paederin is transferred inadvertently from the hands (Fig. 7) [40] (Table 1).

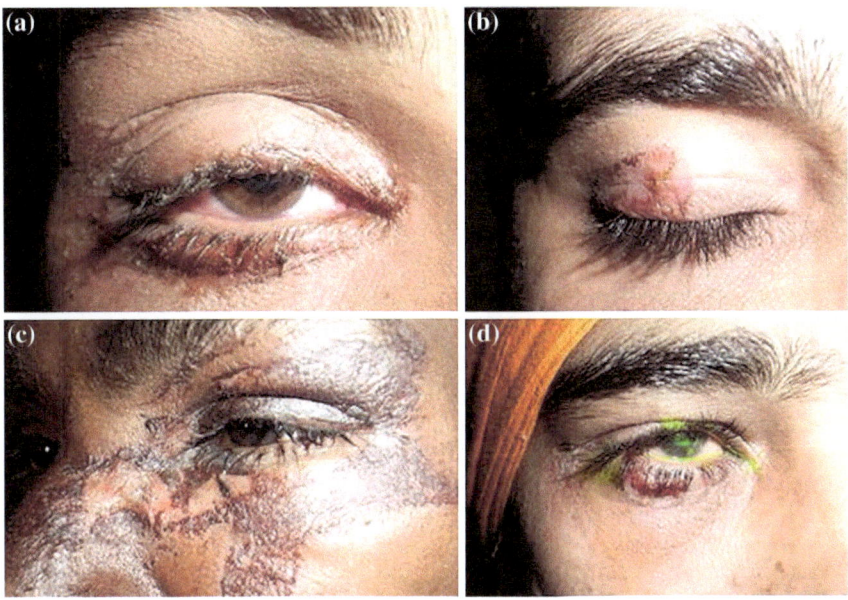

Fig. 7 Ocular involvement in paederus dermatitis. From Prasher, P., Kaur, M., Singh, S. et al. Int Ophthalmol (2017) 37: 885 https://doi.org/10.1007/s10792-016-0352-y

Table 1 Beetles classification

Beetles	Family	Dermatitis mechanism	Caustic substance	Clinical presentation
Order Coleoptera	Oedemeridae (False Blistering Beetle)	Chemical blistering	Cantharidin	· Non-inflammatory · Vesiculobullous
	Meloidiae (Blistering Beetle)	Chemical blistering	Cantharidin	· Non-inflammatory · Vesiculobullous
	Dermestidae (Carpet, Hide, or Larder Beetles)	Hypersensitivity	None but reaction can occur to larval hairs	· Pruritic · Urticarial or papulopustular
	Staphylinidae (Rove Beetles)	Irritant Contact	Paederin	· Inflammatory · Papulovesicular or papulopustular

Bees and Wasps

The order hymenoptera consists of 100,000 species and includes the families Apidae (honey bees), Bombidae (bumble bees), Vespidae (wasps), and Formicidae (ants). Generally known for their painful stings, these insects have long been feared by humans. Most have two pairs of membranous wings with a narrow stalk (petiole) that separates the thorax and abdomen ("wasp waist"). Both bees and wasps are generally social creatures that often congregate in large nests and will attack humans or other animals when they feel that the nest or individual insect is threatened [10, 44].

The stings are caused by females via a modified ovipositor or egg laying apparatus [10]. This can result in an immediate hypersensitivity reaction involving burning pain and an intense erythematous wheal at the site that will subside in several hours [44]. This "wheal and flare" reaction is related to histamine release, dilation of local blood vessels, and increased vascular permeability [10]. More extensive local reactions that can last as long as seven days can occur with swelling and induration measuring several inches in diameter [45, 46]. These are likely due to venom-specific IgE antibodies in sensitized people, which can be identified through skin puncture tests performed with dilute venom to measure any specific circulating IgE [44, 45]. The cell-mediated immune response is also likely responsible for these large local reactions [45].

It is crucial to remove the stinger that may be left in the skin as the venom will continue to seep out. This task can be accomplished by using a dull blade or credit card running nearly parallel to the surface of the skin to dislodge the stinger. Tweezers should be avoided given the risk of compression of the venom sac, which would result in additional venom being injected into the skin [44, 47]. Cool compresses, mild analgesics, and oral antihistamines can be helpful. Additionally, shake lotions such as calamine or other lotions to which powder is added to increase the surface area of evaporation can provide symptomatic relief [48]. For extensive local reactions, systemic steroids may also be beneficial [44, 46, 47].

Severe systemic reactions are an important consideration with regards to the order hymenoptera. Anaphylaxis occurs in 0.3–3% of the population, commonly in men less than 20 years old and presents as urticaria, angioedema, and bronchospasm. This is a potentially fatal reaction which may have no clinical predictors other than prior antigenic exposure. Timely treatment with epinephrine, as well as glucocorticoids and antihistamines, is crucial [46]. The patient should be evaluated in the emergency room as there is a risk for a late phase reaction as other inflammatory mediators continue to be synthesized; a severe systemic reaction can manifest hours later. Early treatment with corticosteroids may help to dampen these delayed effects [47]. Venom immunotherapy may play a role for patients with known allergies and has been shown to decrease the risk of both systemic and large local reactions and to significantly increase disease-specific quality of life [49].

Although likely an underestimate, approximately 50 deaths occur each year due to systemic allergic reactions [10]. Death may also occur after massive envenomation from multiple insect stings causing venom toxicity. For honey bee venom, the estimated LD50 (amount of venom sufficient to kill 50 percent of a population within a certain time) is 19 stings per kilogram of body weight, which translates to approximately 500 stings for a child and 1100–1400 stings for an adult [10]. There has been a case report of massive envenomation that resulted in rhabdomyolysis, vasculitis, and multi-organ failure [50].

Honey Bees

Honey bees are part of the family Apidae. They are remarkably social creatures and tend to live together in hives. The honeybees are known for their unique communication through dancing movements that alert other hive members to food sources [51]. They are unique amongst this group as they are the only species that leave their stinger behind, whereas the other hymenoptera can sting repeatedly [10]. After a sting, the barbed ovipositor of the honey bee remains in the skin while the insect dies due to evisceration. The stinger should be removed carefully without squeezing the area as the attached musculature can continue to pump venom into the skin if left behind (as previously discussed) [52]. Honey bee venom contains vasoactive substances like histamine, melittin (detergent polypeptide), apamin (neurotoxic polypeptide), and enzymes such as phospholipase A2, hyaluronidase, and acid phosphatase [10].

In the US, Africanized honey bees or "killer bees" are more aggressive than native honey bees. While there is no difference in venom, they can mount large attacks that can result in multiple stings and systemic toxicity [10, 46]. Initially introduced in Brazil for crossbreeding with European honey bees (Apis mellifera mellifera) to increase honey production, they escaped and found their way to Texas, Arizona, New Mexico, and California, and they continue to spread into the mid-temperate regions of the US (Fig. 8) [10, 53].

Colony collapse disorder (CCD) is characterized by a sudden unexplained death of a colony of honeybees, particularly the European honeybee (Apis mellifera). It was first reported in the 2000s in the United States, but based on further investigation, previous occurrences prior to this time period may have gone unnoticed. Some commercial beekeeping operations reported up to 50–90% loss of their colonies with an estimated 33% average total annual colony loss across the country. The cause of this condition is unknown, but it may affect the bees' navigational ability, so they do not return after they have left the hive to scavenge for pollen. Several proposed etiologies include pathogens, pesticides, or other stressors that may affect the bees, so there is now a renewed focus on supporting bee colony health as a preventative measure against this phenomenon [54].

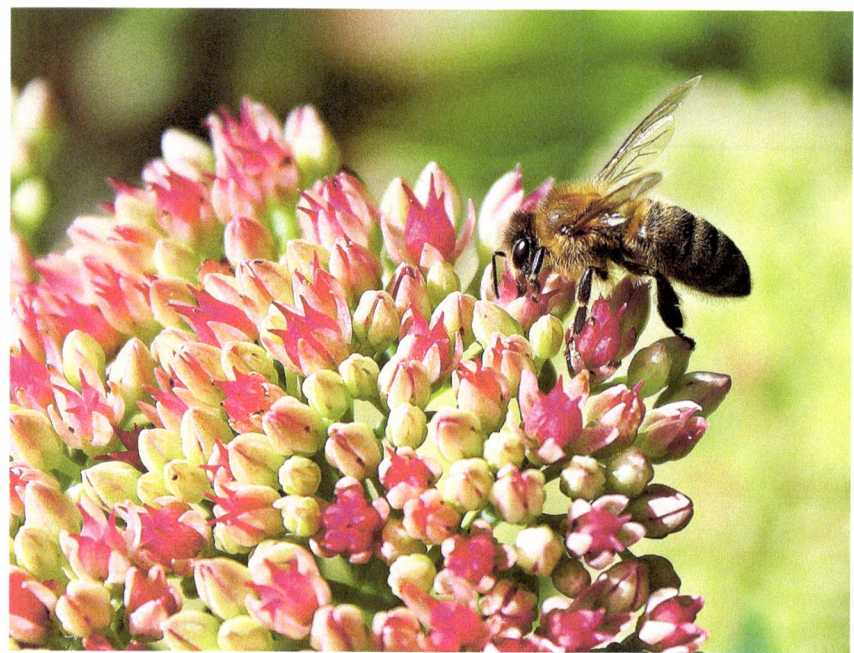

Fig. 8 Honeybee. By Pixabay https://www.pexels.com/photo/bee-bloom-blossom-flora-51936/

Wasps, Hornets, and Yellow Jackets

The family Vespidae includes wasps, hornets, and yellow jackets. Wasps are divided into solitary and social varieties, with the latter living in colonies. While many wasps are solitary, the social wasps include both hornets and yellow jackets. They have segmented antennae, smooth bodies, biting mouthparts, and commonly have wings. Yellow jackets derive their name from their characteristic black and yellow bands on their abdomen (Fig. 9), whereas the hornets are mostly black with some yellow markings on the face, thorax, and abdomen [55].

Unlike the honeybees, the vespids can sting multiple times as their stingers are not barbed, and they can incite severe allergic reactions. The venom is composed of phospholipase, hyaluronidase, and protein antigen 5. In this group, yellow jackets are the principal cause of allergic reactions. They are attracted by food and garbage, and they may emerge during lawn mowing or other outdoor activities when their nests are disturbed. Yellow jackets (Vespula) have underground nests while the nests of the common wasp (Polistes fuscatus) are usually attached to building eaves [46].

On histopathology, most arthropod sting reactions have similar findings with focal spongiosis and dyskeratosis with necrosis or ulceration at the punctum site. Papillary dermal edema and superficial and deep perivascular infiltrate with lymphocytes and eosinophils can be seen. Sometimes pieces of the arthropod can be

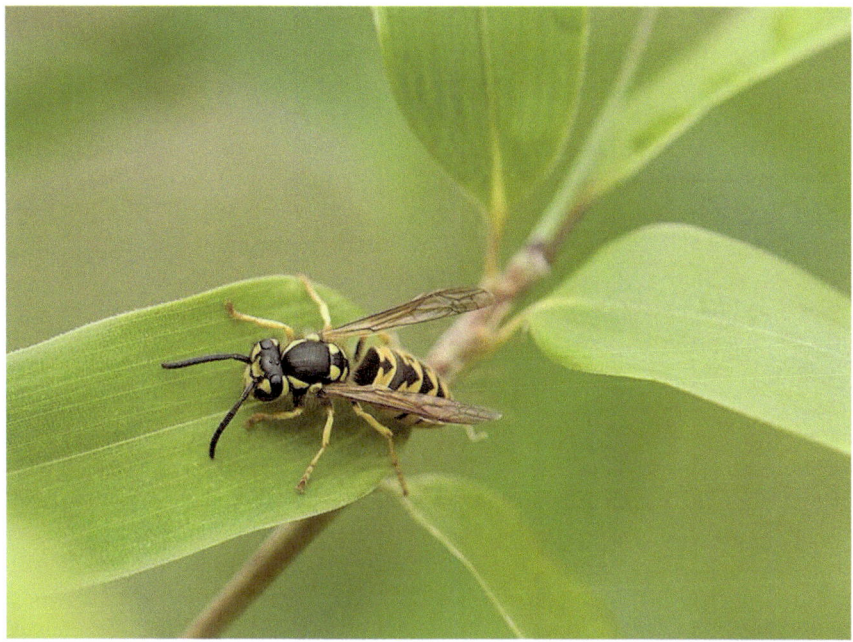

Fig. 9 Yellow jacket. By Pixabay https://www.pexels.com/photo/close-up-insect-leaves-macro-158313/

seen under the microscope, and the foreign materials may precipitate a granulomatous type reaction [47].

Ants

Ants (Formicidae) , like the bees and wasps, are part of the order hymenoptera. Unlike their counterparts, they lack the wings necessary for flight. In North America, they are often viewed as pests. However, ants are actually beneficial for the environment and ecosystem. There are species within this family that can cause significant dermatologic reactions [10].

Fire Ants

The red imported fire ant (Solenopsis invicta) is renowned for its profoundly painful stings that are often featured in pop culture and the media. Originating in Brazil, they were introduced into the US near Alabama in the 1930s and can currently be found in many parts of the southeastern US, especially along the Gulf

Coast [10, 46]. They are usually red or yellow in color and about 1–5 mm in length (Fig. 10). The nest appears as a loose mound with open areas used for ventilation. Ants communicate both through chemical secretions and stridulation, the act of producing sounds by rubbing their body parts together [56].

Their cytotoxic venom contains solenopsin A, which inhibits nitric oxide synthase and degranulates mast cells [5, 57]. The alkaloids within the venom do not seem to generate an IgE antibody response [58]. However, the proteins within the venom, which makes up <10% of the venom by weight, can induce an IgE response in some susceptible people [5]. The ant attaches itself to the skin using its jaw and then pivots around its own head in order to administer multiple stings in a circular pattern with a stinger on the abdomen [46, 52].

Several skin reaction patterns have been described in association with the fire ant. The initial "wheal and flare" resolves in approximately 30–60 minutes. A sterile pustule subsequently appears within 24 hours and finally, the epidermis sloughs off over a period of 48–72 hours. Therapy aimed at preventing or treating these pustules has not been successful. Approximately 17–56% of patients will have a large local reaction with pruritic, erythematous, edematous, and indurated lesions that last from 24 to 72 hours [58]. There is also potential for serious infection and even sepsis. Rare reactions such as anaphylaxis (occurring in up to 1% of stings) and eosinophilic fasciitis have also been described [58–60]. Typical reactions can be treated with topical corticosteroids, anesthetic creams, and oral antihistamines. In the rare case of massive envenomation, oral corticosteroids should be considered. Immunotherapy may play a preventative role for anaphylaxis [58, 61].

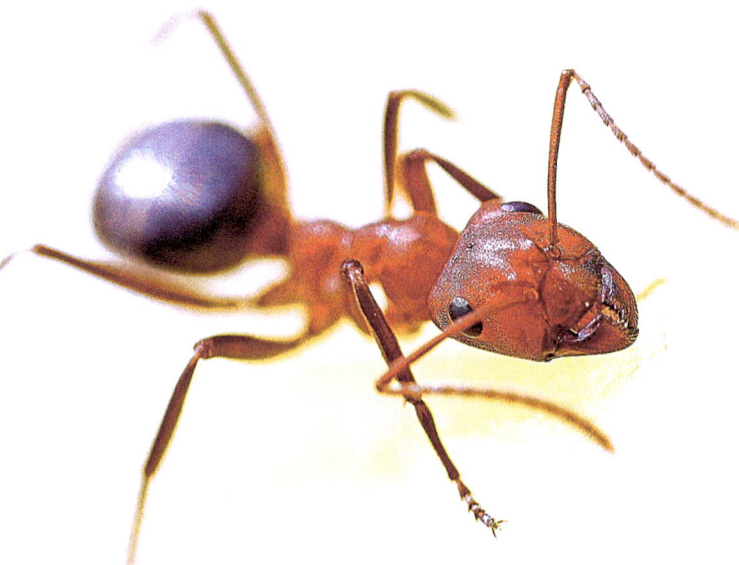

Fig. 10 Fire ant. By Pixabay https://www.pexels.com/photo/nature-red-animal-insect-40825/

Interestingly, Solenopsin, a potent substance that can lead to the inflammatory reactions associated with fire ant dermatitis, is also being studied as a possible treatment for psoriasis in mouse models [62].

References

1. Whitfield JB, Purcell AH. Daly and Doyen's introduction to insect biology and diversity. 3rd edn. Oxford University Press; 2013.
2. Du C, Zhang L, Lu T, et al. Mitochondrial genomes of blister beetles (Coleoptera, Meloidae) and two large intergenic spacers in Hycleus genera. BMC Genom. 2017;18(1):698. https://doi.org/10.1186/s12864-017-4102-y.
3. Blister beetleInsect. Encyclopedia Britannica. https://www.britannica.com/animal/blister-beetle. Accessed 12 Oct 2018.
4. Burnett JW, Calton GJ, Morgan RJ. Blister beetles: "Spanish fly". Cutis. 1987;40(1):22.
5. Haddad V, Cardoso JLC, Lupi O, Tyring SK. Tropical dermatology: venomous arthropods and human skin: part I. Insecta. J Am Acad Dermatol. 2012;67(3):331.e1–e14. https://doi.org/10.1016/j.jaad.2012.04.048.
6. Moed L, Shwayder TA, Chang MW. Cantharidin revisited: a blistering defense of an ancient medicine. Arch Dermatol. 2001;137(10):1357–60. https://doi.org/10.1001/archderm.137.10.1357.
7. Nicholls DSH, Christmas TI, Greig DE. Oedemerid blister beetle dermatosis: a review. J Am Acad Dermatol. 1990;22(5, Part 1):815–19. https://doi.org/10.1016/0190-9622(90)70114-w.
8. Lehmann CF, Pipkin JL, Ressmann AC. Blister beetle dermatosis. AMA Arch Derm. 1955;71(1):36–8.
9. Swarts WB, Wanamaker JF. Skin blisters caused by vesicant beetles. J Am Med Assoc. 1946;131:594.
10. Eldridge BF, Edman J, editors. Medical entomology: a textbook on public health and veterinary problems caused by arthropods. Netherlands: Springer;2000. www.springer.com/us/book/9789401164726. Accessed 12 Oct 2018.
11. Oedemerid beetleInsect. Encyclopedia Britannica. https://www.britannica.com/animal/oedemerid-beetle. Accessed 12 Oct 2018.
12. Arnett R. The false blister beetles of Florida. Tallahassee: Department of Agriculture and Consumer Service Division of Plant Industry. 1984;259:1–3.
13. Christmas TI, Nicholls D, Holloway BA, Greig D. Blister beetle dermatosis in New Zealand. N Z Med J. 1987;100(830):515–7.
14. Herms WB. Ophthalmomyiasis in man due to Cephalomyia (Oestrus) ovis (Linn.). J Parasitol. 1925;12:54–56.
15. Vaurie P. Blistering caused by oedemerid beetles. Coleopt Bull. 1951;5:78–9.
16. Szent-Ivany J, Cletand R. Observations on beetles causing vesicular dermatitis to humans in the territory of Papua and New Guinea. Trans Papua New Guinea Sci Soc. 1966;7:1–8.
17. Fleisher TL, Fox I. Oedemerid Beetle Dermatitis. Arch Dermatol. 1970;101(5):601–5. https://doi.org/10.1001/archderm.1970.04000050105017.
18. Samlaska CP, Samuelson GA, Faran ME, Shparago NI. Blister beetle dermatosis in Hawaii caused by Thelyphassa apicata (Fairmaire). Pediatr Dermatol. 1992;9(3):246–50. https://doi.org/10.1111/j.1525-1470.1992.tb00340.x.
19. Carpet Beetle, HYG-2103-97. https://web.archive.org/web/20010425015704/ http://ohioline.osu.edu/hyg-fact/2000/2103.html. Published 25 Apr 2001. Accessed 11 Mar 2019.
20. Flesh Eating Beetles at the Academy's Skulls Exhibit. https://www.calacademy.org/flesh-eating-beetles. Accessed 11 Mar 2019.

21. Catts EP, Goff ML. Forensic entomology in criminal investigations. Annu Rev Entomol. 1992;37(1):253–72. https://doi.org/10.1146/annurev.en.37.010192.001345.
22. Dermestid beetleinsect. Encyclopedia Britannica. https://www.britannica.com/animal/dermestid-beetle. Accessed 12 Oct 2018.
23. MacArthur KM, Richardson V, Novoa RA, Stewart CL, Rosenbach M. Carpet beetle dermatitis: a possibly under-recognized entity. Int J Dermatol. 2016;55(5):577–9. https://doi.org/10.1111/ijd.12952.
24. Hoverson K, Wohltmann WE, Pollack RJ, Schissel DJ. Dermestid dermatitis in a 2-year-old girl: case report and review of the literature. Pediatr Dermatol. 2015;32(6):e228–33. https://doi.org/10.1111/pde.12641.
25. Ahmed AR, Moy R, Barr AR, Price Z. Carpet beetle dermatitis. J Am Acad Dermatol. 1981;5(4):428–32. https://doi.org/10.1016/S0190-9622(81)70104-X.
26. Cormia FE, Lewis GM. Contact dermatitis from beetles, with a report of a case due to the carpet beetle, Anthrenus scrophulariae. N Y State J Med. 1948;48(18):2037–9.
27. Ayres S, Mihan R. Delusions of parasitosis caused by carpet beetles. JAMA. 1967;199(9):675–675. https://doi.org/10.1001/jama.1967.03120090117036.
28. Ramachandran S, Hern J, Almeyda J, Main J, Patel KS. Contact dermatitis with cervical lymphadenopathy following exposure to the hide beetle, Dermestes peruvianus. Br J Dermatol. 1997;136(6):943–5. https://doi.org/10.1046/j.1365-2133.1997.01828.x.
29. Banney LA, Wood DJ, Francis GD. Whiplash rove beetle dermatitis in central Queensland. Australas J Dermatol. 2000;41(3):162–7. https://doi.org/10.1046/j.1440-0960.2000.00421.x.
30. Senel E, Sahin C. A warmer world means more beetles and more dermatitis. Indian J Occup Environ Med. 2011;15(1):47. https://doi.org/10.4103/0019-5278.82993.
31. Piel J. A polyketide synthase-peptide synthetase gene cluster from an uncultured bacterial symbiont of Paederus beetles. PNAS. 2002;99(22):14002–7. https://doi.org/10.1073/pnas.222481399.
32. Olson PE, Claborn DM, Polo JM, Earhart KC, Sherman SS. Staphylinid (Rove) beetle dermatitis outbreak in the American Southwest? Mil Med. 1999;164(3):209–13. https://doi.org/10.1093/milmed/164.3.209.
33. McGrath L, Piliouras P, Robertson I. Irritant bullous contact dermatitis caused by a rove beetle: an illustrated clinical course. Australas J Dermatol. 2013;54(2):136–8. https://doi.org/10.1111/j.1440-0960.2011.00866.x.
34. Gnanaraj P, Venugopal V, Mozhi MK, Pandurangan CN. An outbreak of Paederus dermatitis in a suburban hospital in South India: a report of 123 cases and review of literature. J Am Acad Dermatol. 2007;57(2):297–300. https://doi.org/10.1016/j.jaad.2006.10.982.
35. Kamaladasa SD, Perera WDH, Weeratunge L. An outbreak of paederus dermatitis in a suburban hospital in Sri Lanka. Int J Dermatol. 1997;36(1):34–6. https://doi.org/10.1046/j.1365-4362.1997.00009.x.
36. Huang C, Liu Y, Yang J, et al. An outbreak of 268 cases of Paederus dermatitis in a toy-building factory in central China. Int J Dermatol. 2009;48(2):128–31. https://doi.org/10.1111/j.1365-4632.2009.03876.x.
37. Al-Dhalimi MA. Paederus dermatitis in Najaf province of Iraq. Saudi Med J. 2008;29(10):1490–3.
38. Awad SS, Abdel-Raof H, Hosam-ElDin W, El-Domyati M. Linear neutrophilic dermatitis: a seasonal outbreak of Paederus dermatitis in Upper Egypt.:5.
39. Turan E. Paederus dermatitis in Southeastern Anatolia, Turkey: a report of 57 cases. Cutan Ocul Toxicol. 2014;33(3):228–32. https://doi.org/10.3109/15569527.2013.834499.
40. Singh G, Ali SY. Paederus dermatitis. Indian J Dermatol Venereol Leprol. 2007;73(1):13. https://doi.org/10.4103/0378-6323.30644.
41. Mokhtar N. Paederus dermatitis amongst medical students in USM. Kelantan. 1993;48(4):4.
42. Poole TRG. Blister beetle periorbital dermatitis and keratoconjunctivitis in Tanzania. Eye. 1998;12(5):883–5. https://doi.org/10.1038/eye.1998.223.

43. Stanimirovic A, Skerlev M, Culav-Košcak I, Kovacevic M. Paederus Dermatitis featuring chronic contact dermatitis. Dermatitis. 2013;24(5):249. https://doi.org/10.1097/DER.0b013e3182948234.
44. Steen CJ, Carbonaro PA, Schwartz RA. Arthropods in dermatology. J Am Acad Dermatol. 2004;50(6):819–42. https://doi.org/10.1016/j.jaad.2003.12.019.
45. Case RL, Altman LC, VanArsdel PP. Role of cell-mediated immunity in Hymenoptera allergy. J Allerg Clin Immunol. 1981;68(5):399–405. https://doi.org/10.1016/0091-6749(81)90139-1.
46. Reisman RE. Insect stings. N Engl J Med. 1994;331(8):523–7. https://doi.org/10.1056/NEJM199408253310808.
47. Steen CJ, Janniger CK, Schutzer SE, Schwartz RA. Insect sting reactions to bees, wasps, and ants. Int J Dermatol. 2005;44(2):91–4. https://doi.org/10.1111/j.1365-4632.2005.02391.x.
48. Souza AD, Strober BE. Chapter 214. Principles of topical therapy. In: Goldsmith LA, Katz SI, Gilchrest BA, Paller AS, Leffell DJ, Wolff K, editors Fitzpatrick's dermatology in general medicine, 8th ed. New York: The McGraw-Hill Companies; 2012. accessmedicine.mhmedical.com/content.aspx?aid=56096360. Accessed 12 Mar 2019.
49. Ludman SW, Boyle RJ. Stinging insect allergy: current perspectives on venom immunotherapy. J Asthma Allergy. 2015;8:75–86. https://doi.org/10.2147/JAA.S62288.
50. Toledo LFM de, Moore DCBC, Caixeta DM da L, et al. Multiple bee stings, multiple organs involved: a case report. Revista da Sociedade Brasileira de Medicina Tropical. 2018;51(4):560–62. https://doi.org/10.1590/0037-8682-0341-2017.
51. Honeybee|insect|Britannica.com. https://www.britannica.com/animal/honeybee. Accessed 11 Apr 2019.
52. Schwartz RA, Steen CJ. Chapter 210. Arthropod Bites and Stings. In: Goldsmith LA, Katz SI, Gilchrest BA, Paller AS, Leffell DJ, Wolff K, editors. Fitzpatrick's dermatology in general medicine, 8th ed. New York: The McGraw-Hill Companies; 2012. accessmedicine.mhmedical.com/content.aspx?aid=56094994. Accessed 8 Oct 2018.
53. McKENNA WR. Killer bees: what the allergist should know. Pediatric Asthma Allergy Immunol. 1992;6(4):275–85. https://doi.org/10.1089/pai.1992.6.275.
54. Colony collapse disorder|Biology|Britannica.com https://www.britannica.com/science/colony-collapse-disorder. Accessed September 4, 2019.
55. wasp|Description, Types, & Facts|Britannica.com. https://www.britannica.com/animal/wasp. Accessed 11 Apr 2019.
56. Fire ant|insect. Encyclopedia Britannica. https://www.britannica.com/animal/fire-ant. Accessed 11 Apr 2019.
57. Yi GB, McClendon D, Desaiah D, et al. Fire ant venom alkaloid, isosolenopsin A, a potent and selective inhibitor of neuronal nitric oxide synthase. Int J Toxicol. 2003;22(2):81–6. https://doi.org/10.1080/10915810305090.
58. deShazo RD, Butcher BT, Banks WA. Reactions to the stings of the imported fire ant. http://dx.doi.org/10.1056/NEJM199008163230707, https://doi.org/10.1056/nejm199008163230707.
59. Stablein JJ, Lockey RF. Adverse reactions to ant stings. Clin Rev Allergy. 1987;5(2):161–75. https://doi.org/10.1007/BF02991205.
60. Mallepalli JR, Quinet RJ, Sus R. Eosinophilic fasciitis induced by fire ant bites. Ochsner J. 2008;8(3):114–8.
61. Stafford CT, Rhoades RB, Bunker-Soler AL, Thompson WO, Impson LK. Survey of whole body-extract immunotherapy for imported fire ant- and other hymenoptera-sting allergy: Report of the fire ant subcommittee of the American academy of allergy and immunology. J Allerg Clin Immunol. 1989;83(6):1107–11. https://doi.org/10.1016/0091-6749(89)90453-3.
62. Arbiser JL, Nowak R, Michaels K, et al. Evidence for biochemical barrier restoration: topical solenopsin analogs improve inflammation and acanthosis in the KC-Tie2 mouse model of psoriasis. Sci Rep. 2017;7(1):11198. https://doi.org/10.1038/s41598-017-10580-y.

Insecta Class: Caterpillars, Butterflies, Moths

Vignesh Ramachandran and Theodore Rosen

Introduction

Lepidoptera, the second largest class of the order *Insecta*, is comprised of moths and butterflies, and their respective caterpillars. Despite over 180,000 recognized organisms within the *Lepidoptera* class, they are largely harmless to humans. Most contact with caterpillars, moths and butterflies is inadvertent. More deliberate exposure may affect children, certain occupational workers (foresters, construction workers), residential gardeners and those entering natural habitats (campers, hikers) [1–5].

Generally, lepidopteran reactions result in nonspecific lesions. As such, the primary cutaneous manifestation and geographical location are most beneficial in making a diagnosis. Lepidopteran reactions may manifest as: (a) localized stinging reactions; (b) papular urticaria and dermatitis; (c) urticarial wheals; (d) hemorrhagic diathesis; (e) dendrolimiasis and pararamose; (f) bites; (g) ophthalmia nodosa; and (h) miscellaneous reactions (Table 1) [6, 7]. "Lepidopterism" is a specific term used to describe systemic illness secondary to harmful effects from direct or airborne contact with caterpillar, cocoon, or moth urticating hairs, spines or body fluids. Symptoms such as diffuse urticaria, conjunctivitis, pharyngitis, headache, nausea, vomiting, wheezing and dyspnea characterize lepidopterism [8, 9].

Species generally causing reactions falling within these categories will be delineated herein along with endemic regions. While most reactions are non-specific, some species cause characteristic lesions which greatly aid clinical suspicion and diagnosis [10].

V. Ramachandran · T. Rosen (✉)
Department of Dermatology, Baylor College of Medicine, Houston, TX, USA
e-mail: rosen@bcm.edu; vampireted@aol.com

V. Ramachandran
e-mail: vigneshr@bcm.edu

© This is a U.S. government work and not under copyright protection in the U.S.;   137
foreign copyright protection may apply 2020
J. Trevino and A. Y-Y. Chen (eds.), *Dermatological Manual of Outdoor Hazards*,
https://doi.org/10.1007/978-3-030-37782-3_10

Table 1 Characterization of moths, butterflies and their respective caterpillars by their dermatologic and systemic manifestations and geographic distribution

Clinical presentation	Organism name (common name)	Geographic distribution
Local stinging reactions		
	Megalopyge opercularis (puss or asp caterpillar)	Mid-Atlantic United States to Central America
	Automeris io (io moth)	Eastern two-thirds United States, southern Canada, Central America
	Hemileuca maia (buck moth)	Eastern United States
	Acharia stimulea (saddleback caterpillar)	Eastern United States to Florida and to Texas
	Uraba lugens (gum leaf skeletonizer moth)	New Zealand (predominantly Greater Auckland region) and Australia
	Thosea penthima (billygoat plum stinging caterpillar)	Australia
	Darna pallivitta (stinging nettle moth)	Southeast Asia
	Dryas iulia (Julia butterfly)	North and South America
Papular urticaria and dermatitis		
	Lymantria dispar (gypsy moth)	Northeast United States and Europe
	Hylesia moths (palometa peluda, the little hairy pigeon)	Caripito, Venezuela
	Orgyia leucostigma (white-marked tussock moth)	Eastern North America to Alberta (Canada) and Texas
	Orgyia pseudotsugata (Douglas-fir moth)	Pacific Northwest (United States and British Columbia, Canada) and California
	Lophocampa caryae (hickory tussock moth)	Northern boundaries of Minnesota and Maine to North Carolina to Texas in southeast/south
	Euproctis chrysorrhoea (brown-tail moth)	Maine and Cape Cod, Massachusetts and Europe (mainly England)
	Lophocampa ingens (tiger moth)	Western United States, including Rocky Mountains
	Arctia caja (garden or great tiger moth)	Northern temperate regions of United States, Canada, and Europe
Urticarial wheals		
	Thaumetopoea wilkinsoni (American pine processionary moth)	Southern Canada to Mexico
	Thaumetopoea pityocampa (European pine processionary)	Coastal regions of north Africa and south Europe
	Thaumetopoea processionea (European oak processionary)	Northern Europe to northern Africa

(continued)

Table 1   (continued)

Clinical presentation	Organism name (common name)	Geographic distribution
Hemorrhagic diathesis		
	Lonomia obliqua and *Lonomia achelous*	South America (predominantly Brazil, Venezuela)
Dendrolimiasis and pararamose		
	Premolis semirufa (Pararama)	Northern Brazil and Amazon region
	Dendrolimus punctatus (Masson pine caterpillar)	East and southeast Asia
Bites		
	Calyptra species	Southeast Asia and eastern Russia
Ophthalmia nodosa	Various, see text section "Ophthalmia Nodosa"	Various, see text sections "Stinging Reactions" to "Ophthalmia Nodosa"

Treatments are generally similar with avoidance and removal of hairs/spines/setae being of utmost importance followed by administration of oral antihistamines and application of topical corticosteroids [7]. Specific treatments will be noted when applicable.

Stinging Reactions

Megalopyge opercularis (Puss or Asp Caterpillar)

In the United States, *Megalopyge opercularis*, also known as the southern flannel moth, inhabits mid-Atlantic states down into the southeast, Texas, and even central America (Fig. 1) [9]. Caterpillars of *M. opercularis*, also known as puss (or asp) caterpillars, live and consume foliage and garden plants [10]. It is one of the most toxic caterpillars in North America and is well-known for severe and painful stings, which most commonly occur between September and October [9]. The puss caterpillar has a long, luxuriant fur-like coat containing venomous spines (Fig. 2).

The classic clinical presentation after contact with pus caterpillar spines consists of grid-like hemorrhagic papules (Fig. 3) [11]. Other symptoms such as burning, pain, swelling, and erythema may also occur [12]. Up to one-third of patients may have systemic symptoms [7, 11–15]. When stings occur near superficial nerves, significant neuropathy may ensue.

Other related *Megalopygidae* (family) species found throughout the United States and Central and South America cause similar stings [16–19].

Treatment is symptomatic. Ice and topical anesthetics can be helpful for mild stings [20]. Severe stings (common with *M. opercularis*) may require oral

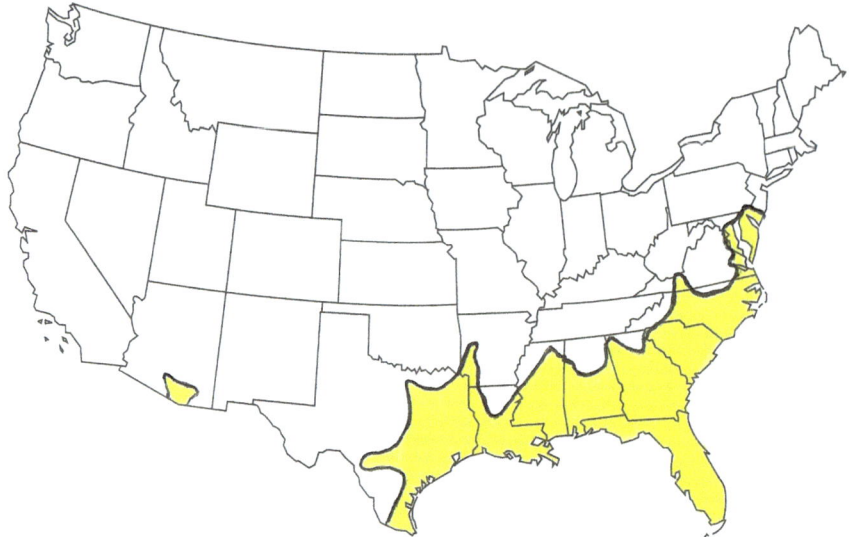

Fig. 1 Geographic distribution of Megalopygidae opercularis (puss or asp caterpillar) in the United States

Fig. 2 Abundant fur-like spines typical of *M. opercularis* caterpillar. (Photo courtesy of Theodore Rosen, MD)

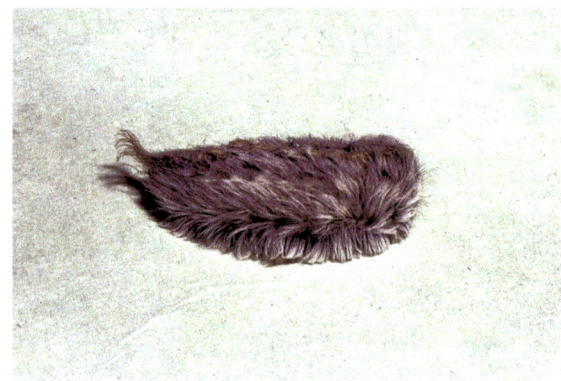

analgesics [11]. Intravenous 10% calcium gluconate solution has also been used successfully [21, 22].

Automeris io (io Moth)

The *Automeris* genus includes over 145 moth species defined by large hindwing eyespots [23]. In the United States, *Automeris io* is the most distinctive species. It is found throughout the eastern two-thirds of the United States (Fig. 4). However,

Fig. 3 Grid-like pattern of hemorrhagic papules typical of *M. opercularis* sting. (Photo courtesy of Theodore Rosen, MD)

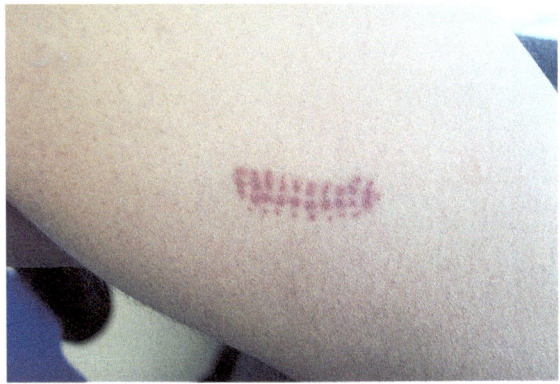

its prevalence is decreasing. Boundaries of its range include southern Canada, west of the Rocky Mountains, and Costa Rica in the south [7, 24, 25]. The io caterpillar is polyphagous, so it may be encountered in any setting with foliage [24]. With maturation, the caterpillar's orange colors evolve to bright green, coupled with longitudinal red and white stripes and venomous spines (Fig. 5) [26].

The caterpillar is well-known for painful stings. However, stings are uncommon. For example, io caterpillar stings were implicated in only 11% of caterpillar stings in Louisiana despite its widespread prevalence in the region [27]. Exposure to cotton and corn crops may result in contact with this caterpillar [28]. Patient description of the caterpillar's distinctive appearance may aid diagnosis [7, 24]. A related species, *A. Louisiana*, is found year-round in Louisiana, Mississippi and the Gulf of Mexico. It also has a larvae capable of stinging [7, 29].

The sting produces an acutely painful and pruritic wheal with erythematous flare (Fig. 6). Chitin particles, each about 10-40 μm, induce an inflammatory response [26]. Pain subsides within a couple of hours and the lesion itself decreases over six-to-eight hours [23, 30]. Systemic sequelae are rare. The venom components are unclassified and general treatments such as oral or injectable antihistamines are ineffective [23, 31].

Hemileuca maia (Buck Moth)

Hemileuca maia, also known as the buck moth, is a member of *Saturniidae* (family). It is found in the eastern United States from Maine to Florida (Fig. 7) [32]. The caterpillars, which emerge in the spring and pupate by late June, feed on oaks [33]. The caterpillar usually has a black body but may be near white on occasion. More characteristic is the abundance of white-to-yellow spots across the thorax and abdomen with rows of multi-branched spines (Fig. 8) [33, 34].

Stings occur after contact with the multi-branched urticating spines. Acute pain is accompanied by tender local lymphadenopathy. Edema and erythema follow

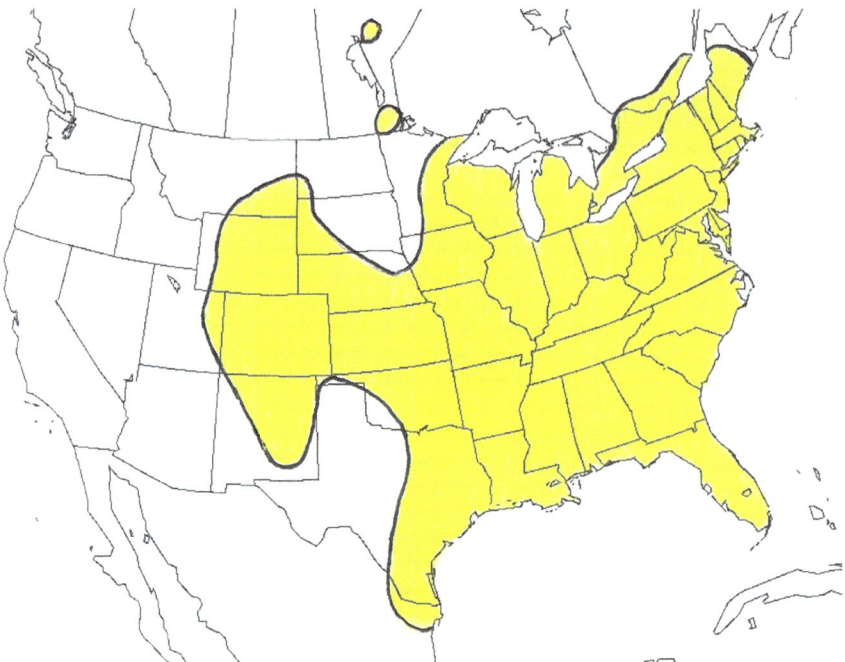

Fig. 4 Geographic distribution of *Automeris io* moth in the United States

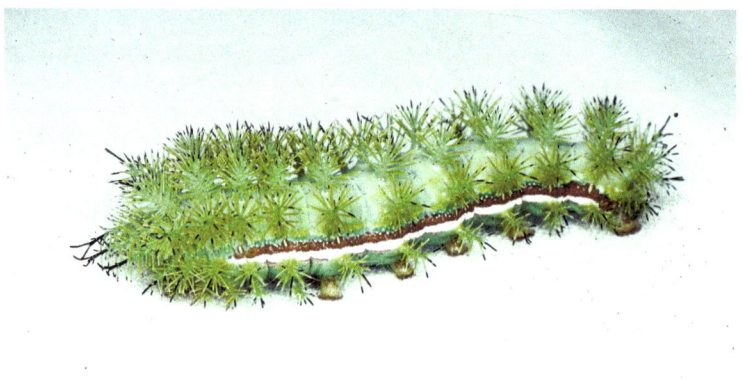

Fig. 5 Characteristic appearance of *Automeris io* caterpillar. (Photo courtesy of Theodore Rosen, MD)

soon thereafter lasting a day to a week [29]. Stinging may be present for up to 10 days with focal pinpoint hemorrhage from sites of spine penetration [34]. This presentation is related to mechanical injury and toxic envenomation from poisonous

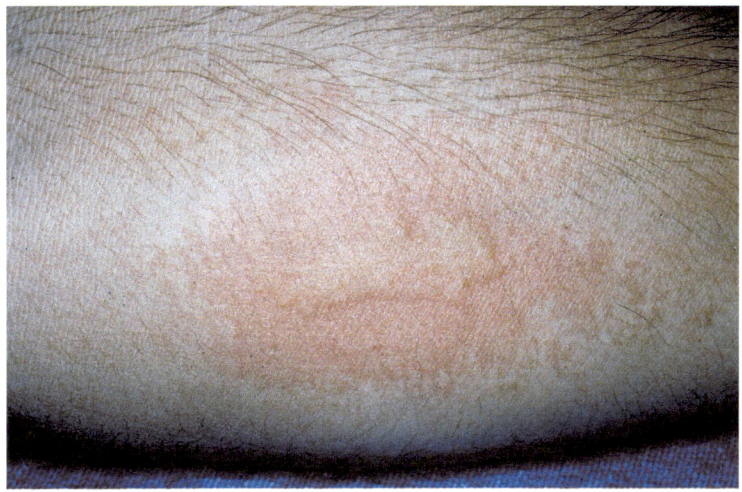

Fig. 6 Acute painful/pruritic wheal following exposure to *Automeris io* caterpillar. (Photo courtesy of Theodore Rosen, MD)

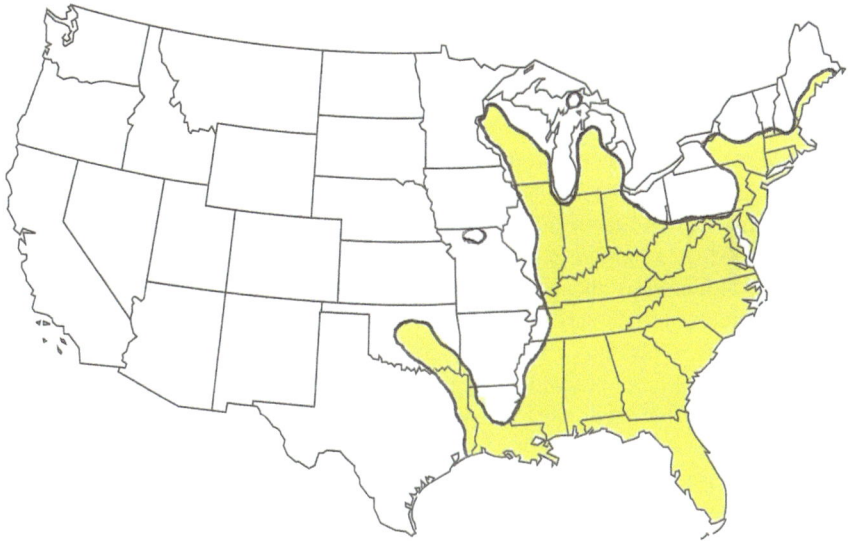

Fig. 7 Geographic distribution of *Hemileuca maia* (buck moth) in the United States

sacs housing venom beneath the spines [35]. Severe reactions to the venom are rare [29, 35]. Diagnosis is made by a combination of history, geographic location and exam. Local compression can be soothing. Avoidance is a must [29].

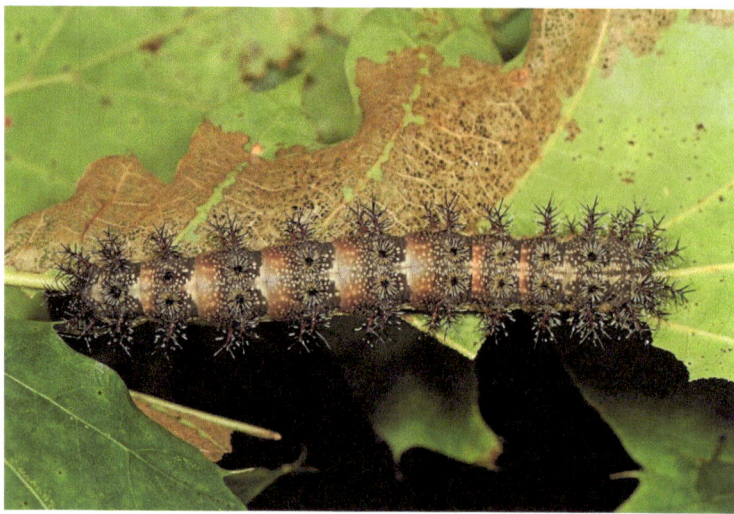

Fig. 8 The buck moth larva demonstrates a characteristic abundance of white-to-yellow spots with rows of multi-branched spines implicated in stings. ("Buck Moth caterpillar—Hemileuca maia, Meadowood Farm SRMA, Mason Neck, Virginia" by Judy Gallagher is licensed under CC BY 2.0)

Acharia stimulea (Saddleback Caterpillar)

Acharia stimulea (formerly *Sibine stimulea*), the saddleback caterpillar, is the best-known caterpillar of the *Limacodidae* family. The caterpillar inhabits the Midwest and eastern United States (Fig. 9). They are mostly found during late summer to October [33]. *A. stimulea* is polyphagous but is more commonly found in bushes (oleander and croton) and palm trees [36]. The saddleback caterpillar has a slug-like appearance (characteristic of *Limacodidae*) with dark brown anterior and posterior surfaces. It also has a vivid aposematic (color schemes and/or markings that serve to warn or repel predators) green midsection (Fig. 10) [7]. The polyphagous caterpillar may be encountered in landscape, agricultural, garden or ornamental foliage. Additionally, reports note agricultural workers handling palm plants are also at increased risk of exposure to the caterpillar [37].

This is one of the most clinically relevant caterpillars in North America. Its large, sturdy spines dispense potent hemolytic venom causing various symptoms [7]. Acute urticaria may occur with anaphylaxis, asthma exacerbations, migraines, gastrointestinal symptoms and a hemorrhagic diathesis [30]. Erythematous, urticarial-to-blistering skin lesions are associated with burning, piloerection and local perspiration [7, 30, 36]. Symptoms typically last less than five hours [10, 30]. However, spines may become airborne, leading to airway hypersensitivity [38].

Diagnosis is based on history of exposure, clinical appearance, occupational risk and geographic location. Removing spines is essential as the longer the spines

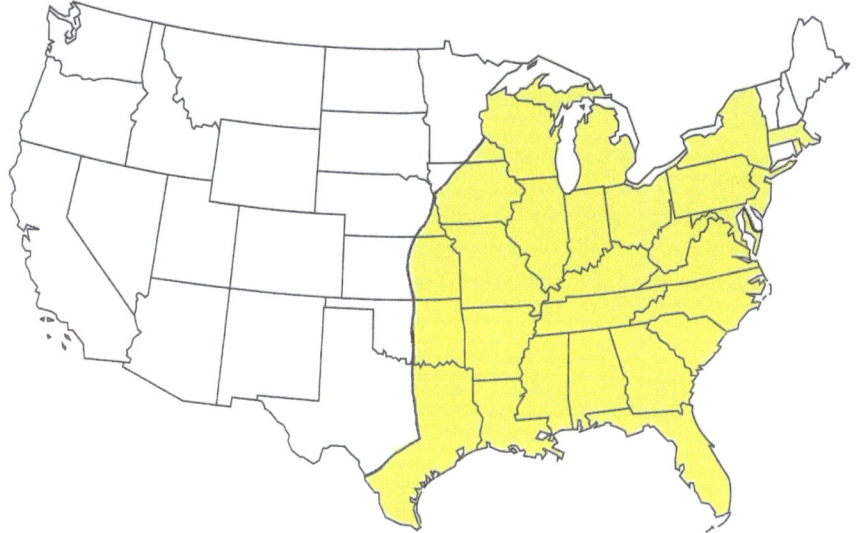

Fig. 9   Geographic distribution of *Acharia stimulea* (saddleback moth) in the United States

Fig. 10   The slug-like
appearing saddleback
caterpillar with characteristic
bright green aposematic
color scheme. ("Saddleback
Caterpillar" by Katja Schulz
is licensed under CC BY 2.0)

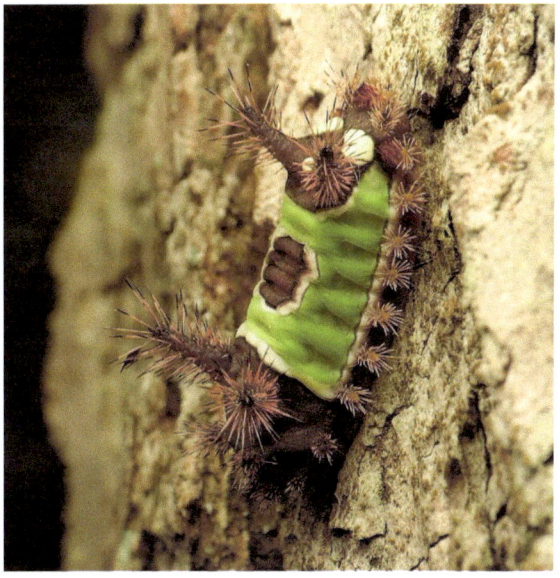

are embedded, the more venom is released, thereby increasing the likelihood of systemic symptoms [7, 30]. Topical steroids improve burning symptoms while antibiotics may prevent superinfection [39]. Protective attire benefits agricultural workers.

Limacodidae (Family) Species

Other *Limacodidae* species are encountered by locals and travelers in Australia and New Zealand.

Uraba lugens (gum leaf skeletonizer moth) is found in the greater Auckland region of New Zealand and parts of Australia [40]. Students in West Auckland have been affected by a pruritic dermatitis characterized by acutely painful sting with erythema and wheals. Lesions resolve within 24–48 hours. [40, 41]. Topical antihistamines may relieve itch [41]. Topical steroids may be beneficial [40, 41].

Australia is also home to *Thosea penthima* (billygoat plum stinging caterpillar). The round, flat, and green-yellow caterpillar produces mild-severe stings due to poisonous spines [7, 42]. Burning pain may occur with localized wheals. One case reports a patient developing crushing chest pain with retrograde radiating arm pain after a sting. Opiate analgesia was needed [42]. Treatment is otherwise symptomatic.

Darna pallivitta (Stinging Nettle Moth)

Native to China, Taiwan, Thailand and other South Asian nations, *Darna pallivitta* established itself in the United States after introduction to the Hawaiian

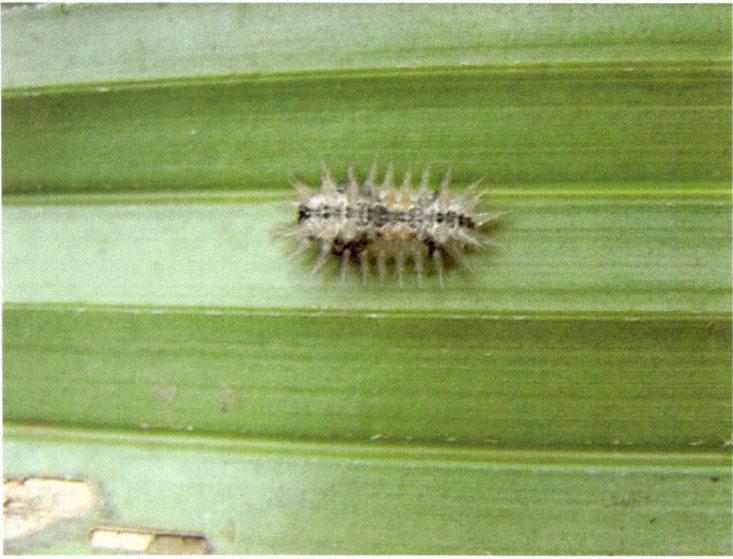

Fig. 11 The stinging nettle moth larva has a dark dorsal stripe and circumferential sharp spines. ("Cocos nucifera (Coconut palm) with Darna pallivitta" by Forest and Kim Starr licensed under CC BY 3.0 US)

Islands in 2001. The caterpillar is polyphagous, consuming various foliage. The white-to-gray caterpillar with a single dark-colored cranial to caudal stripe on the dorsal aspect, is covered by numerous rows of stinging spines (Fig. 11) [43].

The organism is found on residential and commercial landscaping plants, affecting home gardeners, landscapers, and nursery workers. Mechanical injury from spines releases venom which is implicated in the stinging and wheal formation that may last up to five days. Thorough rinsing of the site, oral antihistamines and topical corticosteroid creams may be used [44].

Dryas iulia (Julia Butterfly)

Nymphalidae is one of the largest butterfly families with over 170 species of 42 genera in North America alone. *Dryas iulia* (Julia butterfly), a member of this family endemic to North and South America, is most commonly implicated [45]. In nature, the butterfly is commonly found at the outskirts of forests and woodlands feeding on the nectar of various flowers (Fig. 12). They are popular in conservatories due to their long lifespans and rapid flight during the day [46]. As such, encounters with humans are common. The caterpillar's spines release chemicals causing the dermatitis, which is poorly documented in the literature [29, 46].

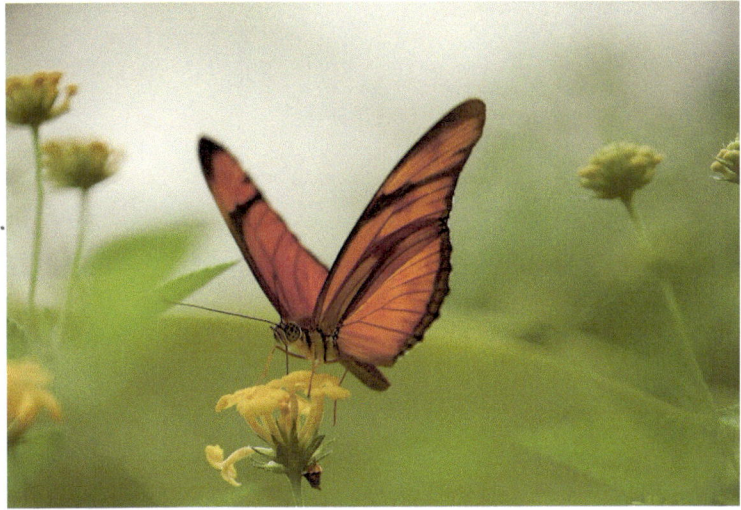

Fig. 12 A Julia butterfly, with orange wings complemented by black accents and a yellow body, drinks the nectar from a flower. ("Dryas Julia" by Böhringer Friedrich is licensed under CC BY-SA 2.5)

Papular Urticaria and Dermatitis

Lymantria dispar (Gypsy Moth)

Lymantria dispar, also known as the gypsy moth, was brought to the United States from Europe around 1869 to develop a silkworm industry. However, after escaping laboratory containment, it inhabited the northeastern United States (Fig. 13) [10]. Its caterpillar consumes leaves of various deciduous trees, most commonly oaks [47]. Most prodigious between May and June, they are identified by their characteristic appearance (Fig. 14). The adult moth may cause deforestation (Fig. 15) [32].

The gypsy moth caterpillar causes a non-specific rash on exposed skin [10]. The pruritic eruption may be papular, urticarial, or eczematous; it resolves over four to seven days (Fig. 16) [48, 49]. Systemic symptoms are uncommon. However, workers raising gypsy moth caterpillars may develop rhinitis, eye irritation, and shortness of breath [47, 50]. Gypsy moth dermatitis is seasonal and parallels expansion of the insect population in the spring. Reduced rainfall allows rapid expansion of the gypsy moth caterpillar population by inhibiting the growth of a natural insect-destroying fungus, *Entomophaga maimaiga*, which translates to an increased adult moth population.

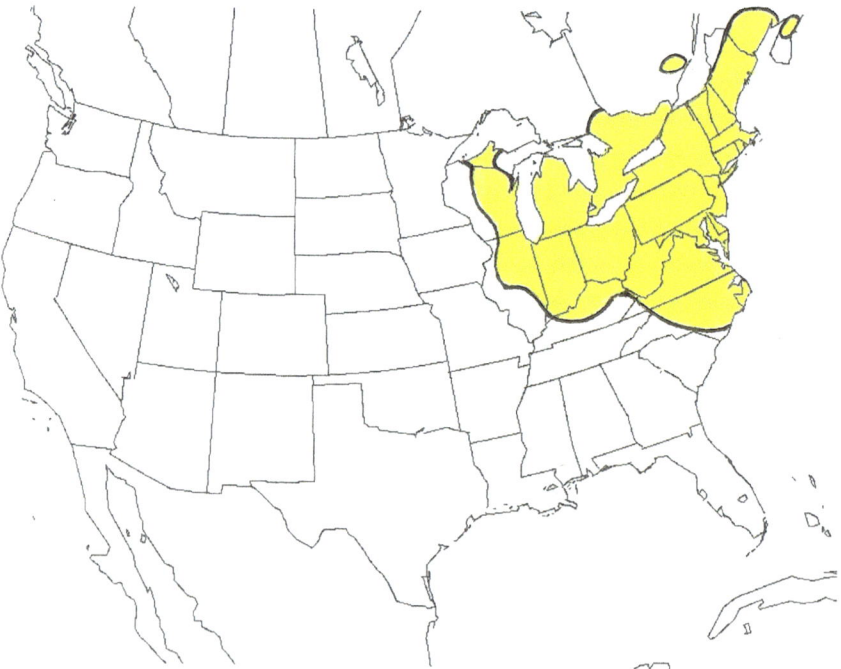

Fig. 13 Geographic distribution of Lymantria dispar (gypsy moth) in the United States

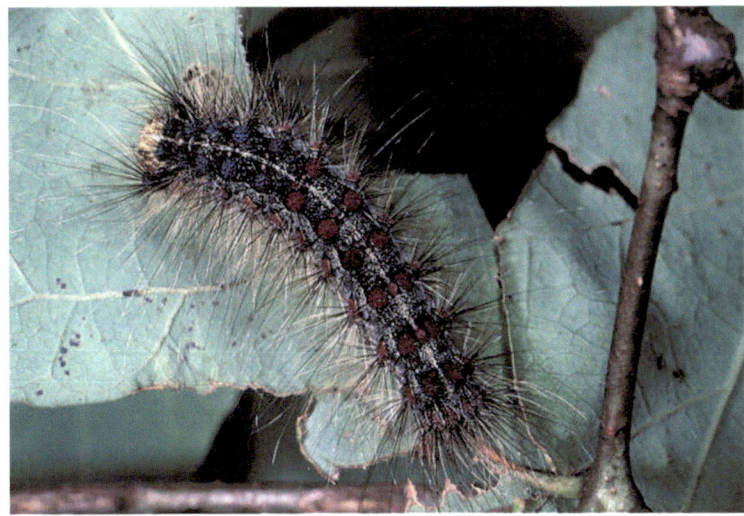

Fig. 14 The caterpillar of the gypsy moth with characteristic paired blue and red protrusions along the dorsal surface with light and dark body hairs. ("Gypsy moth caterpillar" by U.S. Fish and Wildlife Service Headquarters is licensed by CC BY 2.0)

Fig. 15 The adult gypsy moth is well-disguised amidst the foliage of deciduous trees. ("Gypsy Moth" by Ben Sale licensed under CC BY 2.0)

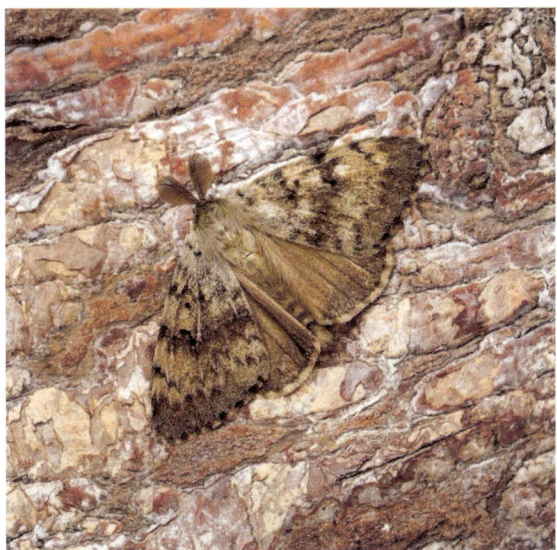

Pathophysiology involves mechanical irritation by hairs, injection of vasoactive substances, like histamine, into the skin and hypersensitivity reactions [47, 48, 51]. One epidemiologic study demonstrated that 79% of patients do not recall direct contact with gypsy moth caterpillars on affected areas, most commonly

Fig. 16 Seasonal non-specific, papular eruption due to gypsy moth caterpillars on Cape Cod. (Photocourtesy of Amy Koff, MD, Cape Cod, Massachusetts)

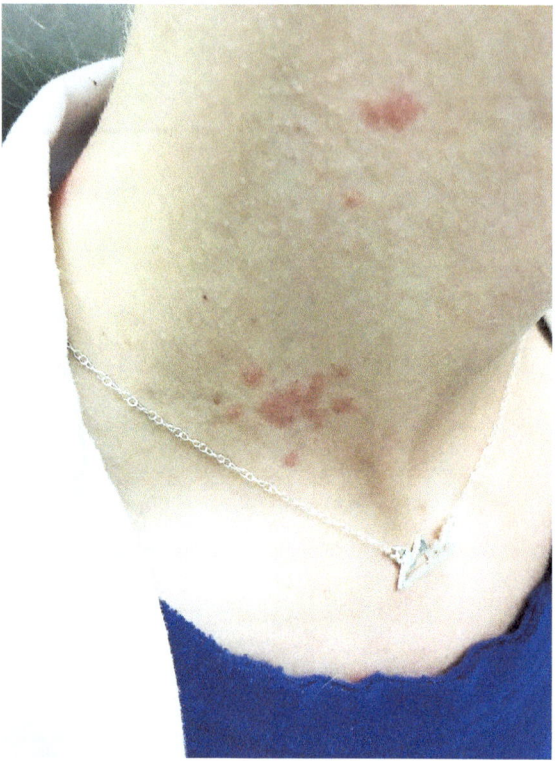

the neck and arms [52]. This has led to speculation that dermatological manifestations may also be due to airborne contact with venomous hairs. Hair removal via tape followed by topical corticosteroids and/or oral antihistamines is recommended [52].

Hylesia Moths (Palometa Peluda, The Little Hairy Pigeon)

The *Hylesia* genus was first implicated in dermatologic conditions in 1918 [53]. Since then, several reports of dermatologic disease have been documented [54]. Endemic to South America, most reports of eruptions occur at the port of Caripito, Venezuela. In fact, the condition is called "Caripito itch" by sailors. In the region, the moth is referred to as *palometa peluda,* or "little hairy pigeon" (Fig. 17) [55, 56]. Urticating hairs found only on the female moths are implicated in clinical manifestations. Dermatoses from *Hylesia moths* are also reported in the United States [54]. These cases are related to travelers returning from voyages to Caripito, Venezuela and have occurred at ports in Boston, Massachusetts and Lake Charles, Louisiana [54, 56, 57].

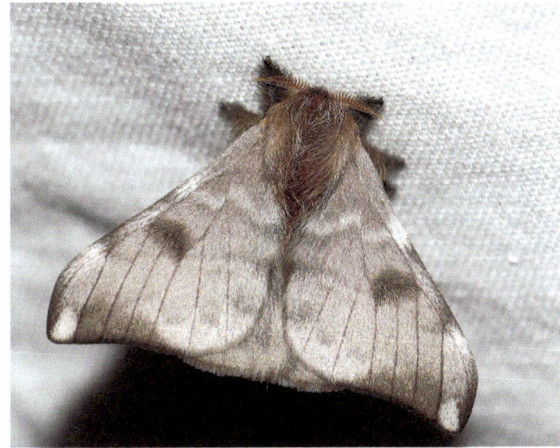

Fig. 17 Fine hairs adorn the body of *Hylesia* moths leading to their moniker "little hairy pigeon". ("Piste de Bélizon, Roura, French Guyana, FRANCE" by Benard DUPONT is licensed under CC BY-SA 2.0)

Minutes to hours after contact with urticating hairs, an intensely pruritic papulourticarial cutaneous eruption occurs with resolution in one week. While mechanical trauma can cause irritation and localized rashes, toxin injection (from abdominal segments 4–7 of females) is implicated in the intensely pruritic cutaneous manifestations [54]. Diagnosis requires a thorough history of travel to the endemic region. Transparent tape stripping can reveal the hairs [51]. Topical and systemic treatments are reportedly unsuccessful. Isolation from further contact results in resolution [54].

Orgyia leucostigma (White-Marked Tussock Moth), Orgyia pseudotsugata (Douglas-Fir Tussock Moth), and Lophocampa caryae (Hickory Tussock Moth)

Orgyia leucostigma (Fig. 18), the white-marked tussock moth, is an *Eribidae* (family) moth common in eastern North America, but its range may extend to Texas, California, and Alberta, Canada. The caterpillars feed on various deciduous and coniferous trees in wooded areas [33]. It is a known pest of shade or fruit trees in urban environments and is implicated in deforestation of Christmas tree plantations [29]. Skin contact with the caterpillar or the cocoon results in a non-specific erythematous, papulourticarial eruption thought to be secondary to the urticating hairs and venom [29, 58, 59].

Closely related to the white-marked tussock moth is *O. pseudotsugata*, or the Douglas-fir tussock moth, which inhabits the Pacific Northwest of the United States and British Columbia, Canada [2]. However, its range has expanded and outbreaks have occurred as far south as southern California [60]. The caterpillar is diffusely covered in white hairs projecting from red tubercles [61]. Caterpillar contact results in welts or a papulourticarial rash. [62–64]. Timber and forestry

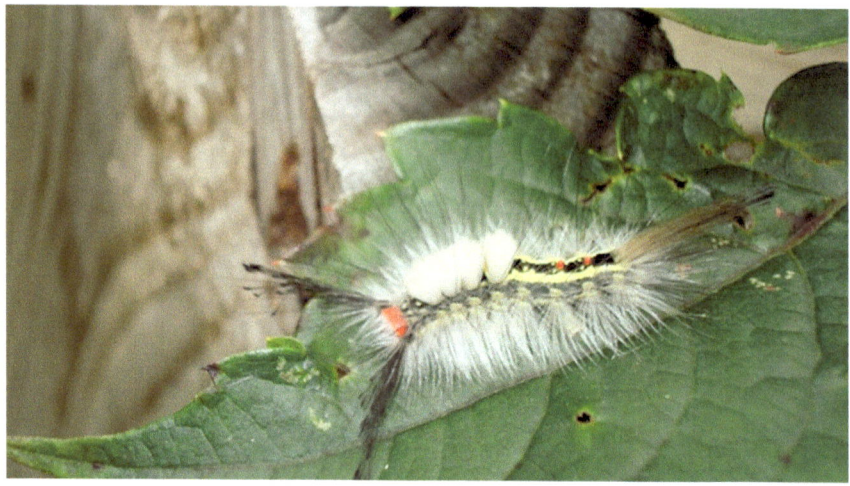

Fig. 18 The white-marked tussock moth larva has a vividly characteristic appearance with white-gray tufts, and a bright red head. ("Caterpillar of the White-marked Tussock Moth" by Treezum is licensed under CC BY-SA 3.0)

workers in the Pacific Northwest are at highest occupational risk. Associated symptoms may include eye itch, rhinorrhea, cough, and respiratory difficulty [64].

Another tussock moth, *Lophocampa caryae* (hickory tussock moth) (Fig. 19), is found in Minnesota and Maine, to the south as far as North Carolina, and to the southwest into Texas [33]. The caterpillar and cocoon are implicated in dermatologic sequelae.

Eggs are laid on foliage, including hickory, ash, elm, pecan and walnut [33]. Contact with the caterpillar causes a mildly pruritic self-resolving eruption [7]. Eighty percent of reports (92.1% dermal exposures, 7.5% oral, and 0.4% ocular) involve children. Treatment (removing spines, irrigation, oral antihistamines and/ or corticosteroids) results in rapid resolution, often within 24 hours [65]. Oral exposure can result in dramatic drooling, anorexia, irritability and require laryngoscopy bronchoscopy/endoscopy [66]. Related caterpillar species (e.g. spotted tussock moth) can cause anaphylaxis [67].

Euproctis chrysorrhoea (Brown-Tail Moth)

Euproctis chrysorrhoea, also known as the brown-tail moth, is the most frequent cause of lepidopteran reactions in England. It was brought to the United States on roses imported from Holland [68]. Its habitat includes coastal Maine and Cape Cod, Massachusetts [69]. It has an affinity for fruit trees but may also be found on elm, oak, hawthorn and blackthorn trees [70]. The hairy, brown caterpillar emerges between April and June (Fig. 20) [70–72].

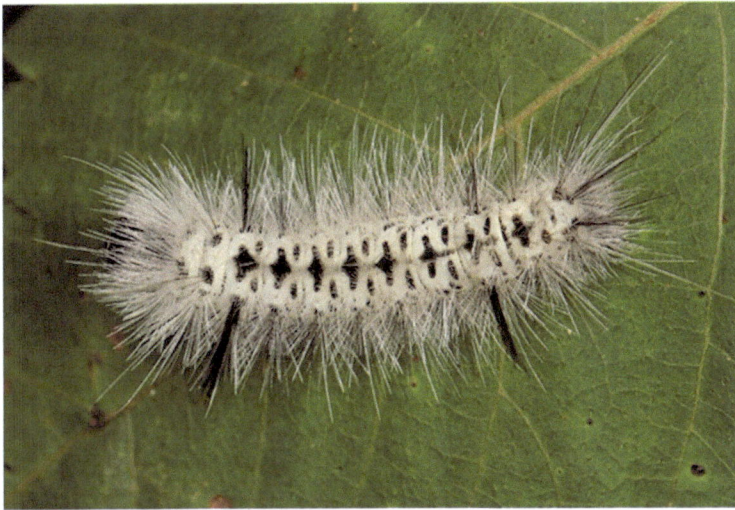

Fig. 19 The caterpillar of the hickory tussock moth with its abundant hair-like setae and characteristic four long black hair pencils. ("Hickory Tussock Moth caterpillar—Lophocampa caryae, Richard Thompson Wildlife Management Area, Linden, Virginia" by Judy Gallagher is licensed under CC BY 2.0)

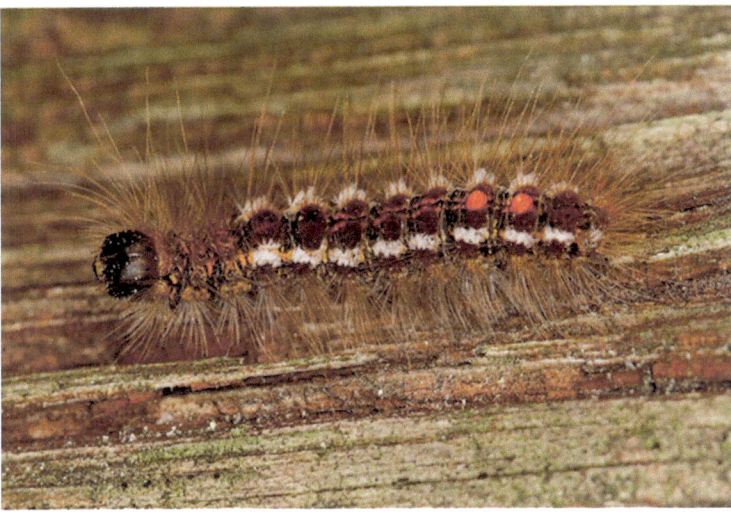

Fig. 20 The browntail moth larva can be identified by its symmetric pair of dorsolateral white stripes and two bright red spots present caudally. ("Eine Raupe des Goldafters Euproctis chrysorrhoea im Burgenland" by spacebirdy is licensed under CC BY-SA 3.0)

The caterpillar is an agricultural and human hazard [69]. The dermatitis is secondary to direct contact or indirect contact with airborne hairs. Patients develop a range of non-specific rashes, including eczematous dermatitis to papular urticaria (most common) to urticarial wheals and vesiculopustular eruptions [7]. Overall, these rashes last from a few hours to several days. Severe cases may even take weeks to resolve. Associated symptoms include bruising, conjunctivitis, rhinitis, ophthalmia nodosa and even anaphylaxis due to high systemic toxin exposure [3, 71, 73, 74].

The rash is thought to be due to a chemical reaction to toxins and mechanical irritation from embedded hairs. Various compounds such as histamines, hydrolases, hemolytic compounds and kallikrein-like serine esterase are released from the caterpillar hairs [5, 75–77].

Patients with systemic symptoms should receive oral antihistamines and non-resolving rashes can benefit from topical steroids [7].

Lophocampa ingens (Tiger Moth) and Arctia caja (Garden or Great Tiger Moth)

Lophocampa ingens, also known as the tiger moth, is a species of *Arctiidae* (family) and is predominantly found in the western United States, including the Rocky Mountain region [78]. Native pines are the hosts. The larvae appear as small, dark and hairy gregarious caterpillars (Fig. 21) [79]. Most exposures uniquely occur in the winter [78].

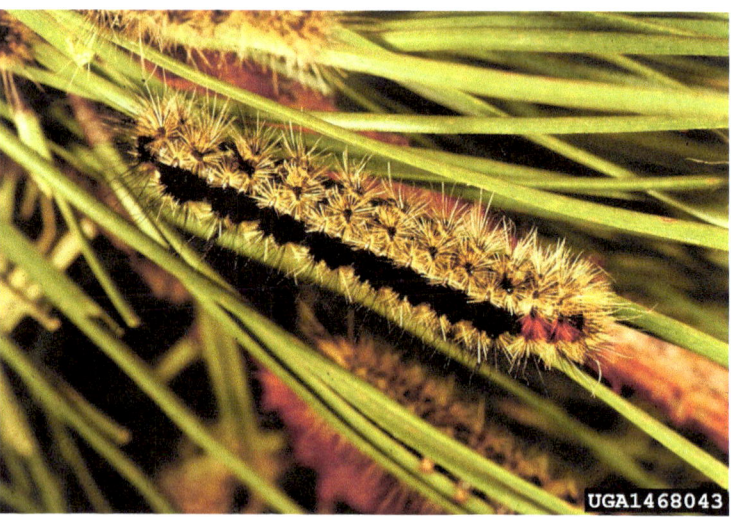

Fig. 21 The tiger moth larva displays vibrant gold markings contrasting upon its black body. The red lateral projections may also aid in identification. ("Lophocampa ingens" by USDA Forest Service is licensed under CC BY 3.0 US)

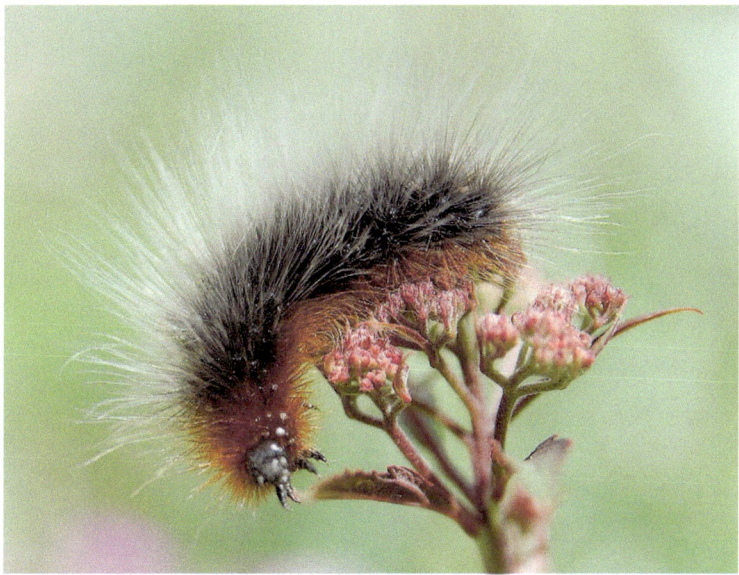

Fig. 22 Fuzzy hairs (owing to the moniker "woolly bears") that are orange-red in color may denote a great tiger moth caterpillar. ("Arctia caja" by Luc Viatour is licensed by CC BY-SA 3.0)

Contact with tiger moths causes a mild papular and pruritic dermatitis [7, 33]. Furthermore, species endemic to South Asia (e.g. *Asota caricae*, tropical tiger moth) are implicated in febrile illness. Chemical characterization of caterpillar and adult moth fluids and chitinous scales in these species reveal highly toxic compounds with inflammatory properties, which are likely the cause of the febrile response [80].

Another species, *Arctia caja* (garden or great tiger moth), is found in northern regions of the United States, Canada, and temperate European regions [79]. The polyphagous organism prefers foliage containing alkaloids [81]. The larval form is covered with fuzzy hair, leading to the moniker "woolly bears" (Fig. 22). The adult moths display bright aposematic beige and orange with black spot color scheme on its wings intended to scare predators. The larval form hatches at the end of the summer, overwinters and re-emerges in the spring [78, 79]. The rash may be caused by the caterpillar or adult moth form. It is self-resolving and described as a non-specific pruritic, erythematous, scaly and papular eruption [17, 18].

Urticarial Wheals

Thaumetopoea Species (Processionary Caterpillars)

Thaumetopoea are commonly implicated in dermatologic conditions: *T. wilkinosoni, T. pityocampa* (together, the pine processionary), and *T. processionea* (oak

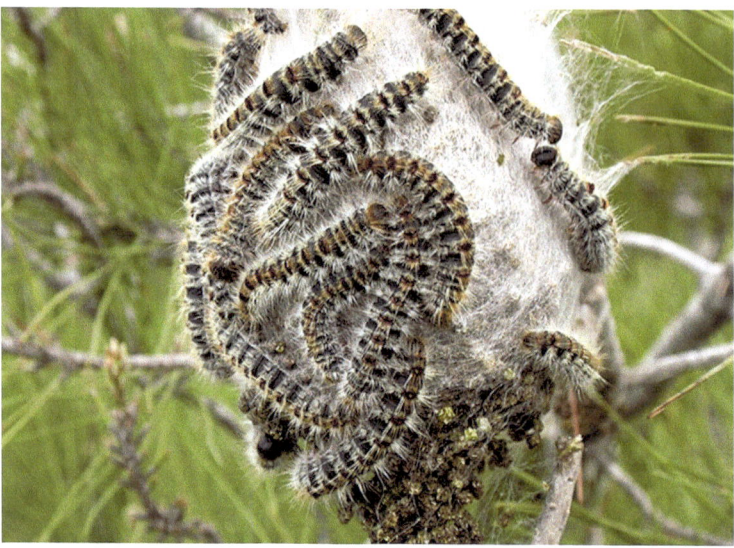

Fig. 23 Processionary caterpillars, such as the Thaumetopoea pityocampa larvae displayed here, are inclined to form long "processions" or rows and have similar color patterns. ("Larva of Thaumetopoea pityocampa from Cyprus" by John H. Ghent, USDA Forest Service, United States is licensed under CC BY 3.0 US)

processionary) [7]. These caterpillars create pheromone trails that result in head-to-tail group travel in a processionary fashion. All the caterpillars are gray-black with raised red-brown tubercles and dense, diffuse hairs of varying color by species (Fig. 23) [29].

T. wilkinsoni, the American pine processionary, is broadly found from southern Canada to Mexico. It is also found in Cyprus, Israel and Turkey. *T. pityocampa* (European pine processionary) inhabits coastal regions of North Africa and southern Europe. *T. processionea* (European oak processionary) can be found from northern Europe to northern Africa [29, 82]. All species may cause outbreaks and deforestation [7].

Dermatitis is due to direct contact (nests, caterpillar, cocoon, or adult moth) or indirect contact (airborne hairs). Lesions can be localized or multifocal. Eruption occurs within 1–12 hours of contact and can present as macules or urticarial papules, although vesicles and bulla are also possible [83]. Pruritus is common [84]. Children allowing the organism to crawl atop their skin may have lesions in linear or meandering configurations [85]. Primary lesions resolve over three to four days [83]. Systemic manifestations, including anaphylaxis, occur in up to 40% of patients [86]. Ten percent of all cases have ocular manifestations (ophthalmia nodosa or blepharoconjunctivitis) [87]. Intraocular disease may result in keratitis, uveitis, or pan-ophthalmitis. Respiratory disease can rarely occur [84, 85]. Treatment is supportive with systemic steroids used in severe cases.

Hemorrhagic Diathesis

Lonomia Species

Endemic of Brazil, Venezuela and other South American nations, *Lonomia obliqua* and *Lonomia achelous* cause a severe and life-threatening disease called Lonomism. These caterpillars are among the deadliest in the world [88]. *L. obliqua* was implicated in 354 deaths between 1989 and 2005 (1.7% fatality rate) [89]. They are brightly- colored caterpillars with multifocal branching spines (Fig. 24) [7].

Contact causes envenomation, resulting in initially mild to severe burning pain. In the next few days, cutaneous, mucosal and visceral hemorrhage occurs, the latter of which is due to venom-related consumption coagulopathy [90, 91]. Death from intracranial hemorrhage or hemorrhage of other organs has been reported [92–95]. Other systemic symptoms include headache, nausea, vomiting and diarrhea. Treatment includes supportive care and anti-venom, which is available in endemic countries [96].

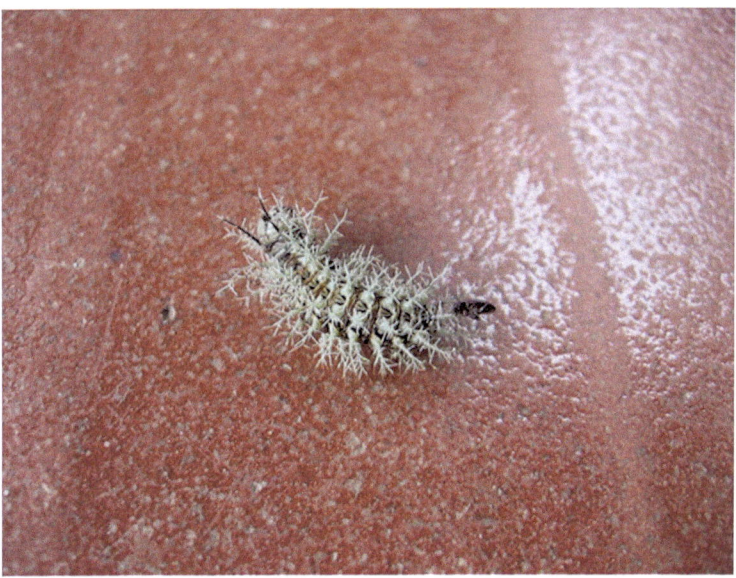

Fig. 24 The light-colored multifocal branching spines of *Lonomia obliqua* caterpillars are characteristic of this potentially deadly species

Dendrolimiasis and Pararamose

Dendrolimus punctatus (Masson Pine Caterpillar) and Premolis semirufa (Pararama)

East Asia is home to many moths, the caterpillars of which may be responsible for human disease. *D. punctatus* is one such moth. Its larval form is implicated in a characteristic well-documented systemic disease, dendrolimiasis, in China, Japan, and other Asian countries [97]. The species itself is a pest causing severe defoliation of young plantations [98]. The organism can be identified by its characteristic silver-gray and black alternating bands throughout its body with lateral-projecting hairs (Fig. 25) [7, 99].

Contact with the caterpillar or cocoon, which is also coated with hairs, results in a non-specific pruritic maculopapular or urticarial eruption. Dendrolimiasis, the systemic illness, may follow. In up to two-thirds of patients with the self-limited eruption, peripheral monoarticular or polyarticular arthritis or chondritis may occur. This may progress to a chronic form resulting in joint destruction. Chondritis may affect the costal, thyroid, and auricular cartilage. Ophthalmitis and scleritis have also been documented [97, 100, 101]. Treatment is supportive.

Premolis semirufa (known colloquially as "Pararama"), found in northern Brazil and the Amazonian region causes an illness similar to dendrolimiasis [87, 102]. Occupational exposure is reported in rubber plantation workers [86].

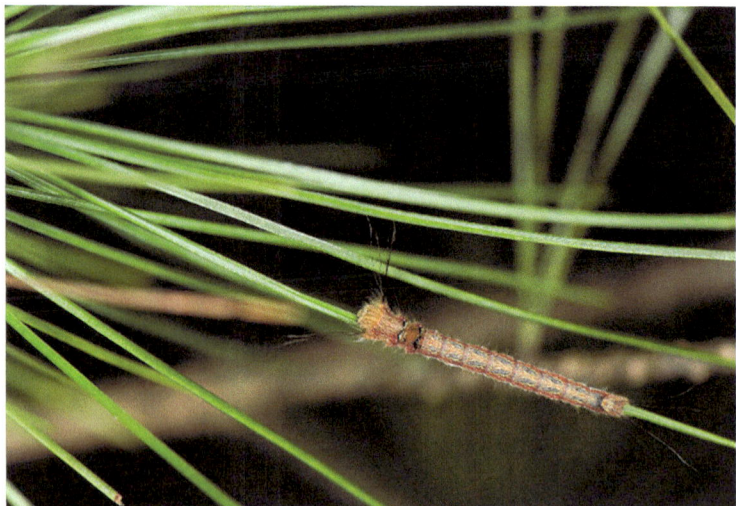

Fig. 25 The slender Masson pine caterpillar has a characteristic silver-gray to bronze-silver and black alternating bands throughout its body. ("Dendrolimus punctatus (Walker, 1855) 馬尾松枯葉蛾" by LiCheng Shih is licensed under CC BY 2.0)

Bites

Calyptra (Biting Moths)

Moths of the genus *Calyptra* are found in the United States, southeastern Asia and eastern Russia (Fig. 26). Not all species under *Calyptra* are able to feed on human blood and documented cases of bites have only occurred in species endemic to Asia and Russia [103, 104].

Male moths bite using a rasp-like proboscis which penetrates uncovered skin. The bites may or may not be painful. Treatment is symptomatic [104].

Ophthalmia Nodosa

Some caterpillar hairs may cause ophthalmia nodosa, secondary to allergic or toxic irritation to the eyes. Contact of hair could be the result of airborne, transfer (from hands or fomites), or direct contact with caterpillar setae [105]. The upper eyelid is most often affected causing chemosis and foreign body sensation. Granulomas may form [7]. Additional sequelae include iritis, vitritis, retinitis and endophthalmitis [106, 107]. Rarely, the optic nerve can be involved [108]. If ophthalmia nodosa is suspected, the patient requires prompt referral to an ophthalmologist for management.

Fig. 26 The *Calyptra* moths, such as *Calyptra orthograpta*, display a remarkable camoflouge scheme disguising them as leaves. ("Calyptra orthograpta" by LiCheng Shih is licensed under CC BY 2.0)

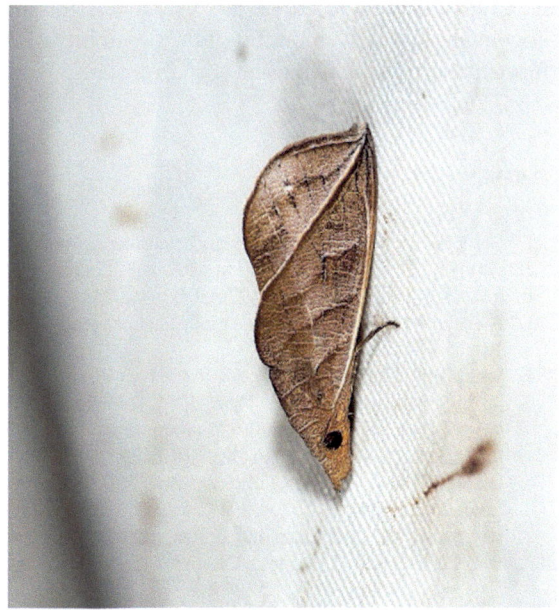

Other Reactions

Oral exposure to caterpillars, butterflies or moths is rarely reported. When this occurs, children are typically involved. Symptoms include drooling, lip irritation, anorexia, pruritus, erythema, pain and dysphagia. While the tongue and lips are most commonly affected, deeper structures in the oral cavity may also be involved due to ingestion of organisms or cocoons [7]. Setae must be removed. Triple endoscopy (direct laryngoscopy, bronchoscopy, esophagoscopy) may be required [66].

Conclusion

Lepidopteran reactions are the result of contact with moths, butterflies and caterpillars. They manifest as a range of dermatologic conditions [10]. This chapter presents common causative organisms.

While many reactions are non-specific and difficult to diagnose, it is important to consider lepidopteran reactions in the differential diagnosis of an appropriate clinical presentation. Avoidance of exposure, removal of hairs/spines and symptomatic treatment (often with antihistamines and corticosteroids) are paramount [7].

Caterpillars are most commonly associated with lepidopteran reactions, usually due to toxic and mechanical irritation. Adult moths and butterflies are much less commonly implicated.

Although thought to be extremely rare in the past, systemic symptoms resulting from contact with moths, butterflies and caterpillars appear to be more common than previously believed [29]. This emphasizes the need for clinicians and outdoor enthusiasts to be mindful of the possibility of these reactions and the need for further investigation regarding such exposures.

References

1. Garty BZ, Danon YL. Processionary caterpillar dermatitis. Pediatr Dermatol. 1985;2(3):194–6.
2. Perlman F, Press E, Googins JA, Malley A, Poarea H. Tussockosis: reactions to Douglas fir tussock moth. Ann Allergy. 1976;36(5):302–7.
3. Alexander S. The browntail moth, its caterpillar and their rash. Clin Exp Dermatol. 1980;5(2):261.
4. Smith WD. Contact urticaria due to the brown-tail moth. Practitioner. 1966;196(175):690–4.
5. de Jong MC, Bleumink E, Nater JP. Investigative studies of the dermatitis caused by the larva of the brown-tail moth (Euproctis chrysorrhoea Linn.) I. Clinical and experimental findings. Arch dermatological Res. 1975;253(3):287–300.
6. Hossler EW. Caterpillars and moths. Part I. Dermatologic manifestations of encounters with Lepidoptera. J Am Acad Dermatol. 2010;62(2):1–10.
7. Hossler EW. Caterpillars and moths. Part II. Dermatologic manifestations of encounters with Lepidoptera. J Am Acad Dermatol. 2010;62(1):13–28.

8. Müller CSL, Tilgen W, Pföhler C. Caterpillar dermatitis revisited: lepidopterism after contact with oak processionary caterpillar. BMJ Case Rep. 2011;2011.
9. Paniz-Mondolfi AE, Pérez-Alvarez AM, Lundberg U, Fornés L, Reyes-Jaimes O, Hernández-Pérez M, et al. Cutaneous lepidopterism: dermatitis from contact with moths of Hylesia metabus (Cramer 1775) (Lepidoptera: Saturniidae), the causative agent of caripito itch. Int J Dermatol. 2011;50(5):535–41.
10. Rosen T. Caterpillar dermatitis. Dermatol Clin. 1990;8(2):245–52.
11. McGovern JP, Barkin GD, McElhenney TR, Wende R. Megalopyge opercularis. JAMA. 1961;175(13):1155.
12. Eagleman DM. Envenomation by the asp caterpillar (Megalopyge opercularis). Clin Toxicol. 2008;46(3):201–5.
13. Stipetic ME, Rosen PB, Borys DJ. A retrospective analysis of 96 "asp" (Megalopyge opercularis) envenomations in Central Texas during 1996. J Toxicol Clin Toxicol. 1999;37(4):457–62.
14. Bishopp F. The puss caterpillar and the effects of its sting on man. United States Dep Agric Dep Circ. 1923;288:1–4.
15. Neustater BR, Stollman NH, Manten HD. Sting of the puss caterpillar: an unusual cause of acute abdominal pain. South Med J. 1996;89(8):826–7.
16. Ardao MI, Sosa Perdomo C, Pellaton MG. Venom of the Megalopyge urens (Berg) caterpillar. Nature. 1966;209(5028):1139–40.
17. Henwood BP, MacDonald DM. Caterpillar dermatitis. Clin Exp Dermatol. 1983;8(1):77–93.
18. Scott H. Stinging caterpillars. Pest Control. 1964;32:24–5.
19. Auerbach PS, Cushing TA, Harris NS. Auerbach's wilderness medicine. 7th ed. Philadephia: Elsevier; 2016.
20. Pinson RT, Morgan JA. Envenomation by the puss caterpillar (Megalopyge opercularis). Ann Emerg Med. 1991;20(5):562–4.
21. Holland DL, Adams DP. "Puss caterpillar" envenomation: a report from North Carolina. Wilderness Environ Med. 1998;9(4):213–6.
22. Micks DW. Clinical effects of the sting of the "puss caterpillar" (Megalopyge opercularis S & A) on man. Tex Rep Biol Med. 1952;10(2):399–405.
23. Hossler EW, Elston DM, Wagner DL. What's eating you? Io moth (Automeris io). Cutis. 2008;82(1):21–4.
24. Tuskes PM, Tuttle JP, Collins M. The wild silk moths of North America. Ithaca: Cornell University Press; 1996.
25. Manley T. Diapause, voltinism, and foodplants of Automeris io (Saturniidae) in the southeastern United States. J Lepid Soc. 1993;47(4):303–21.
26. Battisti A, Holm G, Fagrell B, Larsson S. Urticating hairs in arthropods: their nature and medical significance. Annu Rev Entomol. 2011;56(1):203–20.
27. Everson GW, Chapin JB, Normann SA. Caterpillar envenomations: a prospective study of 112 cases. Vet Hum Toxicol. 1990;32(2):114–9.
28. Stratton-Porter G. Moths of the Limberlost. Loschberg: Jazzybee Verlag; 1921.
29. Diaz JH. The evolving global epidemiology, syndromic classification, management, and prevention of caterpillar envenoming. Am J Trop Med Hyg. 2005;72(3):347–57.
30. Hossler EW. Caterpillars and moths. Dermatol Ther. 2009;22(4):353–66.
31. Hughes G, Rosen T. Automeris io (caterpillar) dermatitis. Cutis. 1980;26(1):71–3.
32. Covell CV. A field guide to moths of eastern North America. 2nd ed. Martinsville: Virginia Museum of Natural History; 2005.
33. Wagner DL. Caterpillars of Eastern North America: a guide to identification and natural history. Princeton: Princeton University Press; 2005.
34. Baldwin, JL, Hall M et al. Insect pest 2012 management guide. Louisianna State University Agriculture Center. https://www.lsuagcenter.com/~/media/system/4/9/6/c/496c381f03be739dc3d77b0a1a893309/pub1838_2018lainsectpestmgmtguide-pdf.pdf. Accessed 14 Dec 2018.

35. Bessin, R.: University of Kentucky Entomology: stinging caterpillars. 2010. https://web.archive.org/web/20110927135147, http://www.ca.uky.edu/entomology/entfacts/ef003.asp. Accessed 12 Dec 2018.
36. Edwards EK Jr, Edwards EK, Kowalczyk AP. Contact urticaria and allergic contact dermatitis to the saddleback caterpillar with histologic correlation. Int J Dermatol. 1986;25(7):467.
37. Howard FW, Moore D, Giblin-Davis RM, Abad RG. Insects on palms. New York: CABI; 2001.
38. Bibbs, CS, Howard, FJ. Saddleback caterpillar Acharia stimulea (Clemens) (Insecta: Lepidoptera: Limacodidae). 2015. http://entnemdept.ifas.ufl.edu/creatures/. Accessed 13 Dec 2018.
39. Claudet I, Maréchal C. A transatlantic caterpillar. Pediatr Emerg Care. 2009;25(3):186–7.
40. Derraik J. Erucism in New Zealand: exposure to gum leaf skeletoniser (Uraba lugens) caterpillars in the differential diagnosis of contact dermatitis in the Auckland region. N Z Med J. 2006;119(1241):U2142.
41. Derraik JGB. Three students exposed to Uraba lugens (gum leaf skeletoniser) caterpillars in a West Auckland school. N Z Med J. 2007;120(1259):U2656.
42. Isbister GK, Whelan PI. Envenomation by the billygoat plum stinging caterpillar (Thosea penthima). Med J Aust. 2018;173(11–12):654–5.
43. Nagamine WT, Epstein ME. Chronicles of Darna pallivitta (Moore 1877) (Lepidoptera: Limacodidae): biology and larval morphology of a new pest in Hawaii. Pan-Pac Entomol. 2007;83(2):120–35.
44. Chun S, Hara A, Niino-DuPonte R, Nagamine W, Conant P, Hirayama C. Identifying and managing stinging nettle caterpillars. 2005. https://hdoa.hawaii.gov/pi/files/2013/01/npa01-03_netcat.pdf. Accessed 12 Dec 2018.
45. Freitas AVL, Brown KS. Phylogeny of the nymphalidae (Lepidoptera). Syst Biol. 2004;53(3):363–83.
46. Scott JA. The butterflies of North America: a natural history and field guide. 1st ed. Palo Alto: Stanford University Press; 1997.
47. Etkind PH, Odell TM, Canada AT, Shama SK, Finn AM, Tuthill R. The gypsy moth caterpillar: a significant new occupational and public health problem. J Occup Med. 1982;24(9):659–62.
48. Centers for Disease Control (CDC). Rash illness associated with gypsy moth caterpillars–Pennsylvania. MMWR Morb Mortal Wkly Rep. 1982;31(13):169–70.
49. Anderson JF, Furniss WE. Epidemic of urticaria associated with first-instar larvae of the gypsy moth (Lepidoptera: Lymantriidae). J Med Entomol. 1983;20(2):146–50.
50. Wirtz RA. Occupational allergies to arthropods—documentation and prevention. Bull Entomol Soc Am. 1980;26(3):356–62.
51. Shama SK, Etkind PH, Odell TM, Canada AT, Finn AM, Soter NA. Gypsy-moth-caterpillar dermatitis. N Engl J Med. 1982;306(21):1300–1.
52. Kikuchi T, Kobayashi K, Sakata K, Akasaka T. Gypsy moth-induced dermatitis: a hospital review and community survey. Eur J Dermatol. 2012;22(3):384–90.
53. Leger M, Mouzels P. Dermatose prurigineuse determince par des pari lIons saturnides de genre Hylesia. Bull Soc Pathol Exot. 1918;11:104–7.
54. Dinehart SM, Archer ME, Wolf JE, McGavran MH, Reitz C, Smith EB. Caripito itch: dermatitis from contact with Hylesia moths. J Am Acad Dermatol. 1985;13(5 Pt 1):743–7.
55. Wirtz RA. Allergic and toxic reactions to non-stinging arthropods. Annu Rev Entomol. 1984;29(1):47–69.
56. Jourdain F, Girod R, Vassal JM, Chandre F, Lagneau C, Fouque F, et al. The moth Hylesia metabus and French Guiana lepidopterism: centenary of a public health concern. Parasite. 2012;19(2):117–28.
57. Hill WR, Rubenstein AD, Kovacs J. Dermatitis resulting from contact with moths (genus Hylesia). JAMA. 1948;138(10):737–40.
58. Goldman L, Sawyer F, Levine A, Goldman J, Goldman S, Spinager J. Investigative studies of skin irritations from caterpillars. J Invest Dermatol. 1960;34:67–79.

59. Gilmer PM. A comparative study of the poison apparatus of certain lepidopterous larvae. Ann Entomol Soc Am. 1925;18(2):203–39.

60. Coleman TW, Jones MI, Courtial B, Graves AD, Woods M, Roques A, et al. Impact of the first recorded outbreak of the Douglas-fir tussock moth, Orgyia pseudotsugata, in southern California and the extent of its distribution in the Pacific Southwest region. For Ecol Manage. 2014;329:295–305.

61. Natural Resources Canada: Douglas-fir tussock moth. 2015. https://tidcf.nrcan.gc.ca/en/insects/factsheet/1000009. Accessed 14 Dec 2018.

62. Redd JT, Voorhees RE, Török TJ. Outbreak of lepidopterism at a boy scout camp. J Am Acad Dermatol. 2007;56(6):952–5.

63. Hoover AH, Nelson E. Skin symptoms attributed to tussock moth infestation. Cutis. 1974;13:597.

64. Press E, Googins JA, Poareo H, Jones K. Health hazards to timber and forestry workers from the Douglas fir tussock moth. Arch Environ Health. 1977;32(5):206–10.

65. Kuspis DA, Rawlins JE, Krenzelok EP. Human exposures to stinging caterpillar: Lophocampa caryae exposures. Am J Emerg Med. 2001;19(5):396–8.

66. Tripi PA, Lee R, Keiper JB, Jones AW, Arnold JE. An unusual case of ingestion of a moth cocoon in a 14-month-old girl. Am J Otolaryngol. 2010;31(2):123–6.

67. DuGar B, Sterbank J, Tcheurekdjian H, Hostoffer R. Beware of the caterpillar: anaphylaxis to the spotted tussock moth caterpillar. Lophocampa maculata. Allergy Rhinol (Providence). 2014;5(2):113–5.

68. Potter A. Brown-tail moth dermatitis. JAMA. 1909;LIII(18):1463–4.

69. Elkinton JS, Parry D, Boettner GH. Implicating an introduced generalist parasitoid in the invasive browntail moth's enigmatic demise. Ecology. 2006;87(10):2664–72.

70. Frago E, Guara M, Pujade-Villar J, Selfa J. Winter feeding leads to a shifted phenology in the browntail moth Euproctis chrysorrhoea on the evergreen strawberry tree Arbutus unedo. Agric For Entomol. 2010;12(4):381–8.

71. Blair CP. The browntail moth, its caterpillar and their rash. Clin Exp Dermatol. 1979;4(2):215–22.

72. Burgess AF. Imported insect enemies of the gypsy moth and the brown-tail moth. In: United States Department of Agriculture Technical Bulletin. 1929. https://naldc.nal.usda.gov/download/CAT86200081/PDF. Accessed 17 Dec 2018.

73. Hall-Smith PJ, Graham P. Beware the furry caterpillar. Clin Exp Dermatol. 1980;5(2):261–2.

74. Kephart CF. The poison glands of the larva of the brown-tail moth (Euproctis chrysorrhoea Linn.). J Parasitol. 1914;1(2):95.

75. de Jong MC, Kawamoto F, Bleumink E, Kloosterhuis AJ, Meijer GT. A comparative study of the spicule venom of Euproctis caterpillars. Toxicon. 1982;20(2):477–85.

76. Bleumink E, de Jong MC, Kawamoto F, Meyer GT, Kloosterhuis AJ, Slijper-Pal IJ. Protease activities in the spicule venom of Euproctis caterpillars. Toxicon. 1982;20(3):607–13.

77. Kawamoto F, Kumada N. Kininogenase activity and kinin-like substance in the venomous spicules and spines of lepidopteran larvae. Adv Exp Med Biol. 1979;120A:51–5.

78. United States Department of Agriculture. Tiger Moth: tree-top tents appear early in conifers. 2011. https://www.fs.usda.gov/Internet/FSE_DOCUMENTS/stelprdb5320266.pdf. Accessed 17 Dec 2018.

79. The Editors of Encyclopaedia Britannica. Tiger moth [Internet]. Encyclopedia Britannica. 2018 [cited 2018 Dec 15]. p. 1. https://www.britannica.com/animal/tiger-moth.

80. Wills PJ, Anjana M, Nitin M, Varun R, Sachidanandan P, Jacob TM, et al. Population explosions of tiger moth lead to Lepidopterism mimicking infectious fever outbreaks. PLoS ONE. 2016;11(4):e0152787.

81. Rothschild M, Reichstein T, von Euw J, Aplin R, Harman RRM. Toxic lepidoptera. Toxicon. 1970;8(4):293–6.

82. Bruchim Y, Ranen E, Saragusty J, Aroch I. Severe tongue necrosis associated with pine processionary moth (Thaumetopoea wilkinsoni) ingestion in three dogs. Toxicon. 2005;45(4):443–7.

83. Bonamonte D, Foti C, Vestita M, Angelini G. Skin Reactions to pine processionary caterpillar Thaumetopoea pityocampa Schiff. Sci World J. 2013;867431:1–6.

84. Vega JM, Moneo I, Ortiz JCG, Palla PS, Sanchís ME, Vega J, et al. Prevalence of cutaneous reactions to the pine processionary moth (Thaumetopoea pityocampa) in an adult population. Contact Dermatitis. 2011;64(4):220–8.

85. Vega ML, Vega J, Vega JM, Moneo I, Sánchez E, Miranda A. Cutaneous reactions to pine processionary caterpillar (Thaumetopoea pityocampa) in pediatric population. Pediatr Allergy Immunol. 2003;14(6):482–6.

86. Vega JM, Moneo I, Armentia A, López-Rico R, Curiel G, Bartolomé B, et al. Anaphylaxis to a pine caterpillar. Allergy. 1997;52(12):1244–5.

87. Bessler E, Biedner B, Yassur Y. Thaumetopoea wilkinsoni (toxic pine caterpillars) blepharoconjunctivitis. Am J Ophthalmol. 1987;103(1):117–8.

88. Veiga AB, Blochtein B, Guimarães JA. Structures involved in production, secretion and injection of the venom produced by the caterpillar Lonomia obliqua (Lepidoptera, Saturniidae). Toxicon. 2001;39(9):1343–51.

89. Kowacs PA, Cardoso J, Entres M, Novak EM, Werneck LC. Fatal intracerebral hemorrhage secondary to Lonomia obliqua caterpillar envenoming. Arq Neuropsiquiatr. 2006;64(4):1030–2.

90. Arocha-Piñango CL, Guerrero B. [Hemorrhagic syndrome induced by caterpillars. Clinical and experimental studies]. Invest Clin. 2003;44(2):155–63.

91. Zannin M, Lourenço DM, Motta G, Dalla Costa LR, Grando M, Gamborgi GP, et al. Blood coagulation and fibrinolytic factors in 105 patients with hemorrhagic syndrome caused by accidental contact with Lonomia obliqua caterpillar in Santa Catarina, southern Brazil. Thromb Haemost. 2003;89(2):355–64.

92. Chan K, Lee A, Onell R, Etches W, Nahirniak S, Bagshaw SM, et al. Caterpillar-induced bleeding syndrome in a returning traveller. Can Med Assoc J. 2008;179(2):158–61.

93. Chudzinski-Tavassi AM, Carrijo-Carvalho LC. Biochemical and biological properties of Lonomia obliqua bristle extract. J Venom Anim Toxins Incl Trop Dis. 2006;12(2):159–71.

94. Arocha-Piñango CL, de Bosch NB, Torres A, Goldstein C, Nouel A, Argüello A, et al. Six new cases of a caterpillar-induced bleeding syndrome. Thromb Haemost. 1992;67(4):402–7.

95. Portela Gamborgi G, Brett Metcalf E, J.G. Barros E. Acute renal failure provoked by toxin from caterpillars of the species Lonomia obliqua. Toxicon. 2006;47(1):68–74.

96. Da Silva WD, Campos CM, Gonçalves LR, Sousa-e-Silva MC, Higashi HG, Yamagushi IK, et al. Development of an antivenom against toxins of Lonomia obliqua caterpillars. Toxicon. 1996;34(9):1045–9.

97. Huang DZ. Dendrolimiasis: an analysis of 58 cases. J Trop Med Hyg. 1991;94(2):79–87.

98. Billings RF. The pine caterpillar Dendrolimus punctatus in Vietnam; Recommendations for integrated pest management. For Ecol Manage. 1991;39:97–106.

99. Yang C-H, Yang P-C, Li J, Yang F, Zhang A-B. Transcriptome characterization of dendrolimus punctatus and expression profiles at different developmental stages. PLoS ONE. 2016;11(8):e0161667.

100. Lawson JP, Liu YM. Pinemoth caterpillar disease. Skeletal Radiol. 1986;15(6):422–7.

101. Villas-Boas IM, Gonçalves-de-Andrade RM, Pidde-Queiroz G, Assaf SLMR, Portaro FC V., Sant'Anna OA, et al. Premolis semirufa (Walker, 1856) Envenomation, disease affecting rubber tappers of the Amazon: searching for caterpillar-bristles toxic components. PLoS Negl Trop Dis. 2012;6(2):e1531.

102. Costa RM, Atra E, Ferraz MB, da Silva NP, de Souza JM, Batista Júnior J, et al. "Pararamose": an occupational arthritis caused by lepidoptera (Premolis semirufa). An epidemiological study. Rev Paul Med. 1993;111(6):462–5.

103. Zaspel JM, Kononenko VS, Goldstein PZ. Another blood feeder? Experimental feeding of a fruit-piercing moth species on human blood in the primorye territory of far Eastern Russia (Lepidoptera: Noctuidae: Calpinae). J Insect Behav. 2007;20(5):437–51.

104. Bänziger H. Skin-piercing blood-sucking moths II: Studies on a further 3 adult Calyptra [Calpe] sp. (Lepid., Noctuidae). Acta Trop. 1979;36(1):23–37.
105. Watson PG, Sevel D. Ophthalmia nodosa. Br J Ophthalmol. 1966;50(4):209–17.
106. Cadera W, Pachtman MA, Fountain JA, Ellis FD, Wilson FM. Ocular lesions caused by caterpillar hairs (ophthalmia nodosa). Can J Ophthalmol. 1984;19(1):40–4.
107. Steele C, Lucas DR, Ridgway AE. Endophthalmitis due to caterpillar setae: surgical removal and electron microscopic appearances of the setae. Br J Ophthalmol. 1984;68(4):284–8.
108. Fraser SG, Dowd TC, Bosanquet RC. Intraocular caterpillar hairs (setae): Clinical course and management. Eye. 1994;8(5):596–8.

Insecta Class: Flies and Mosquitoes

Kavya Desai and Campbell Stewart

Introduction

Flies and mosquitoes are essential players in the ecosystem; however, they have a significant impact on human health. These insects can be nuisances through their sheer presence and their bite reactions, but most importantly they are vectors for some of the most devastating diseases on the planet. In fact, mosquitoes are considered the deadliest animal on the planet, killing in excess of 700,000 humans each year, mostly through transmission of malaria [1]. This chapter details the specific flies and mosquitoes responsible for these diseases, as well as their prevention and treatment options.

Suborder Nematocera

Family Culicidae

Aedes

Classification of arthropod

Order Diptera, Suborder Nematocera, Family Culicidae, Genus Aedes.

K. Desai
Department of Internal Medicine and Dermatology, The University if Minnesota,
401 East River Parkway, VCRC 1st Floor, Suite 131, Minneapolis, MN 55455, USA
e-mail: desai.45@wright.edu

C. Stewart (✉)
Uconn Health, 21 South Road, Farmington, CT, USA
e-mail: castewart@uchc.edu

© Springer Nature Switzerland AG 2020
J. Trevino and A. Y-Y. Chen (eds.), *Dermatological Manual of Outdoor Hazards*,
https://doi.org/10.1007/978-3-030-37782-3_11

Description of arthropod

Aedes mosquitoes have three sections (head, thorax, and abdomen). The two most common disease causing species of *Aedes* mosquitoes are *Aedes aegypti* and *Aedes albopictus*. The former is a brown/black mosquito with a silver dorsal pattern (lyre-shaped) and black and white striped legs. This species is considered to be the primary vector of yellow fever, dengue fever and chikungunya [2, 3]. These mosquitoes typically bite during the day but are most active around dawn and dusk. The latter is also brown/black with black and white striped legs but has a single silver line on its body. In addition to transmitting dengue and chikungunya, *Aedes albopictus* also transmits West Nile virus, Eastern equine encephalitis, and Japanese encephalitis. *Aedes albopictus* are also daytime biters [4].

Clinical Diseases

Yellow Fever

Transmission

Yellow fever is caused by a Flavivirus transmitted to humans mainly by the *Aedes* spp. mosquitoes (in Africa) or *Haemagogus* spp. and *Sabethes* spp. mosquitoes (in South America) [5]. The incubation period lasts about 3–6 days with symptoms lasting a few days in mild cases and weeks in severe cases. Approximately 5–20% of those infected will develop symptoms [6]. Humans are viremic from just before fever onset up until about 5 days later. Mosquitoes can acquire the virus from humans during this time [7].

Epidemiology

The disease is endemic to Africa, where the incidence is highest in West Africa. Yellow fever is also endemic to South America, where the incidence is much lower but the mortality rate is higher than in West Africa. This is likely due to genetic variations in the host species [5].

Diagnosis

As mentioned previously, not all infected individuals become symptomatic. Of those who are symptomatic there is a wide variation of presentation. Mild cases can be non-specific presenting with fever and headache and resolving after a few days. About 15% of those who are symptomatic progress to a "toxic phase"; these severe cases can include high fever, jaundice, bleeding, hematemesis, shock and multi-organ failure [6, 8]. Very ill patients may have a relative bradycardia in comparison to what is expected with such a high fever, termed Faget's sign. Laboratory abnormalities that can be seen throughout various stages of the disease include leukopenia followed by leukocytosis, hyperbilirubinemia, elevated prothrombin and partial thromboplastic times, reduced platelet count, and elevated serum transaminase levels [9]. Diagnosis is usually based on clinical findings and history, especially in resource-poor settings; however, there are serologic assays for detection of IgM and IgG antibodies. Since there is some cross-reactivity with other viruses (such as dengue), there is a neutralization test that is performed in order to confirm the presence of yellow fever virus. There is also a PCR test that can be performed, but it is not an extremely sensitive test since viral load can be low by the time symptoms are present [6].

As its name suggests, one of the main dermatologic manifestations of yellow fever is jaundice. Cutaneous manifestations have also been reported to occur in response to the yellow fever vaccine. Most commonly, these include injection site reactions, urticaria and anaphylaxis, although there have been rare cases of localized bullous fixed drug eruption and lichen striatus following vaccine administration [10, 11].

Treatment

Since the disease is vaccine preventable, it is preferable to avoid infection through vaccination, especially since most treatment is supportive care. To date there has been no approved antiviral therapy for yellow fever virus and many treatment options are experimental [12]. Correcting hypovolemia, hypoxia, and shock can reduce mortality in patients with severe symptoms [8].

Prevention

The yellow fever vaccine is recommended for individuals traveling to endemic areas. The vaccine is considered safe for individuals over the age of 9 months with the exception of patients who have an egg allergy, are immunosuppressed (medications, cancer, organ transplant, etc.), or are HIV positive with a low CD4+count (typically <200/mm^3) [13]. The vaccine is a live attenuated version of the 17D strain of the virus and is effective for about 10 years [11]. Limiting exposure to mosquitoes and wearing protective clothing/insect repellents can also be beneficial.

Dengue Fever

Transmission

Dengue fever is also caused by a Flavivirus. The incubation period lasts from 3–8 days, followed by a variable symptomatic period, with severe disease lasting 5–6 days.

Epidemiology

While dengue used to be limited to 9 countries around the world, the latter half of the twentieth century saw the spread of the disease to more than 100 countries worldwide (mostly in tropical regions). The disease continues to result in significant morbidity and mortality worldwide with an estimated 500,000 cases severe enough to require hospitalization annually. Countries that experienced outbreaks in 2018 include Bangladesh, Cambodia, India, Myanmar, Malaysia, Pakistan, Philippines, Thailand and Yemen [14].

Diagnosis

There is wide variation in the presentation of patients infected with dengue. Dengue fever is the mildest form of disease. Dengue hemorrhagic fever and dengue shock syndrome are more severe forms of infection. Of note, dengue hemorrhagic fever is more likely in patients who have had multiple exposures to different strains of the dengue virus [8]. In younger children, the illness is usually mild, presenting with a fever and rash. More severe cases are common in adults with high biphasic fever, retro-orbital pain, headache, myalgias, arthralgias, nausea and vomiting [15].

Cutaneous manifestations are quite common in dengue fever, occurring in anywhere from 50 to 82% of patients. The characteristic rash takes a predictable course. Prior to symptom onset, the patient will develop erythematous facial flushing likely due to capillary dilation. This will typically be followed a few days later by a morbilliform eruption which spares the palms and soles. Some patients develop diffuse erythema with white islands of sparing. Some patients will also complain of pruritus with rash onset. As expected, hemorrhagic manifestations (petechiae, purpura, and ecchymosis) are seen with dengue hemorrhagic fever and dengue shock syndrome but are less common in dengue fever. Involvement of the mucosa occurs in approximately 15–30% of cases, predominantly those with the hemorrhagic form. When the eyes are affected, conjunctival and scleral injection can be seen. When oral mucosa is involved, there can be crusting of the tongue and lips as well as vesicles on the palate [15].

Treatment

Supportive care is the mainstay of treatment. Studies have compared the benefit of various interventions to determine optimal treatments for patients with dengue. The most important component of treatment during the critical period is fluid resuscitation. The optimal method of fluid repletion is via oral intake; however, when this is not possible, 0.9% saline is the recommended first line intravenous option. Randomized control trials have shown marginal benefit of using fresh frozen plasma (to increase platelet counts) and nasal CPAP (for improvement of hypoxemia) in certain patient populations [16].

Prevention

The best way to prevent dengue is through vector control and avoidance of mosquitoes. Additionally, early detection of signs and symptoms can be beneficial in treatment. Due to the four distinct serologic subtypes, developing a vaccine which is effective against all forms of dengue has been difficult. Vaccination for dengue remains controversial. A live attenuated vaccine, Dengvaxia® (CYD-TDV), was developed in 2015. Although the vaccine is considered safe in seropositive individuals, some studies have shown that seronegative recipients of the vaccine had higher risk of developing more severe dengue than those seronegative subjects who were unvaccinated. Thus, the WHO recommends exploring risks and benefits based on specific region and available resources [14].

Chikungunya

Transmission

Chikungunya fever is caused by an Arbo virus transmitted to humans mainly by the *Aedes aegypti* and *Aedes albopictus* mosquitoes. The incubation period lasts about 3–7 days, followed by an abrupt onset of symptoms which can last anywhere from 1 to 7 days.

Epidemiology

Epidemics of chikungunya fever have occurred predominantly in tropical regions such as sub-Saharan Africa, southeast Asia, parts of the Indian subcontinent and several islands in the Indian Ocean [17]. The United States has had very few cases of chikungunya over the last few years, and the vast majority has been associated with international travel. In 2018, the CDC reported 90 travel-associated cases and 0 locally-transmitted cases of chikungunya virus in the United States [18].

Diagnosis

Symptoms include high biphasic fever (every 2–6 days) with shaking chills, polyarticular arthritis involving both small and large joints, and a variety of cutaneous manifestations. One study described the cutaneous manifestations of chikungunya fever observed during an outbreak in south India [19]. The most common cutaneous manifestation was hyperpigmented macules distributed on the central face which lasted for about 3 weeks. Other less common cutaneous manifestations include aphthous-like ulcers, lichenoid eruptions, vesiculobullous lesions and vasculitic lesions lasting anywhere from a few days to several weeks. Cutaneous lesions most frequently appear during the symptomatic acute phase of the illness although some patients develop lesions after the fever subsides. Very few patients develop skin lesions more than 1 month after the acute phase. These features vary based on skin type, and are more commonly reported in darker skin types based on the geography and epidemiology of the disease.

Treatment

Treatment for Chikungunya consists of mostly supportive care. Cutaneous lesions are self-resolving and nonsteroidal anti-inflammatory drugs can be used to reduce fever and joint pains.

Prevention

Since no vaccine exists, prevention is mainly by avoidance of mosquitoes. As with most mosquito- transmitted illnesses, it is important to avoid stagnant water, use long sleeve shirts and pants, apply insect repellents (such as DEET) to skin and apply permethrin to clothing [20].

Zika

Transmission

Zika virus is caused by a virus transmitted to humans mainly by the *Aedes aegypti* and *Aedes albopictus* mosquitoes. The incubation period lasts anywhere from 3 to 12 days with symptoms lasting up to a week [21]. The virus can also be transmitted sexually and vertically from a pregnant woman to her fetus, resulting in birth defects [22].

Epidemiology

The Zika virus was first detected in 1947 in monkeys in Uganda and shortly after, it was detected in *Aedes africanus* mosquitoes. Before the early 2000s, there were only about a dozen reported cases of Zika-related illnesses. Beginning in 2007, there were a few outbreaks occurring in the Federated States of Micronesia and French Polynesia. In 2014, a large outbreak in Brazil brought Zika to the forefront of media attention. In the following years, it became more common in the Americas although the only cases of local transmission in the United States have occurred in Florida and Texas [23].

Diagnosis

Common symptoms in adults are nonspecific and include fever, headache, myalgias and arthralgias, rash and conjunctivitis. The rash most commonly appears 3–12 days after initial infection and begins as diffuse macules and papules, typically sparing the palms and soles of the feet. The rash starts on the face and spreads to extremities. On occasion, petechiae and mucosal bleeding in the mouth can occur. The rash will resolve spontaneously after about a week and is difficult to distinguish from the rashes of some of the other diseases (Chikungunya and Dengue Fever) transmitted by the same mosquitoes [21].

Congenital Zika infection has received significant media attention in recent years due to the outbreak in 2015. The Zika Outcomes and Development of Infants and Children (ZODIAC) investigation assessed the growth and development of 19 children (aged 19–24 months) with laboratory evidence of Zika virus infection. Microcephaly is the major birth defect seen in these children, but other findings were seizures, cerebral palsy, motor impairment, pneumonia/bronchitis, sleeping difficulties and impaired response to auditory and visual stimuli [24].

Treatment

Like many other mosquito-borne diseases, the treatment for Zika virus is generally supportive treatment and prevention remains the most important method of control. An important consideration is that if there is a possibility of coinfection by Dengue virus, treatment should avoid NSAIDs and aspirin use due to the possibility of hemorrhage and Reye's syndrome [25].

Prevention

In addition to protection against mosquito bites and vector control, it is also important to realize that this disease can be transmitted sexually and vertically. Barrier methods of contraception or abstinence are effective in reducing sexual transmission [26].

Anopheles

Classification of arthropod

Order Diptera, Suborder Nematocera, Family Culicidae, Genus Anopheles.

Description of arthropod

Anopheles mosquitoes have three sections (head, thorax, and abdomen). A distinguishing feature of these mosquitoes is that their wings have black and white scales. These mosquitoes are most well-known for their transmission of *Plasmodium* parasites to humans which can result in malaria.

Clinical Diseases

Malaria

Transmission

Of the hundreds of species that belong to the *Anopheles* genus, there are only a few dozen which are responsible for the transmission of malaria in many different parts of the world. Only female mosquitoes are capable of transmitting disease. Infected *Anopheles* mosquitoes are responsible for transmission of the

Plasmodium parasite from human to human. Malaria parasites first multiply in the human liver and are released into the bloodstream where they cause systemic manifestations. When a mosquito ingests a blood meal from an infected human, the male and female *Plasmodium* gametocytes are able to mate in the mosquito's body and proliferate. After about two weeks, an infectious form (sporozoite) of the parasite can be found in the salivary glands of the mosquito at which point the cycle can be repeated [27].

Epidemiology

Malaria is a disease which disproportionately affects individuals living in tropical climates. This is because *Anopheles* mosquitoes depend on warm climates to multiply, and parasites are dependent on their vector for transmission. Globally, the highest rates of transmission are found in Sub-Saharan Africa and Southeast Asia. It was estimated that malaria was responsible for around 216 million cases and 445,000 deaths worldwide in 2016. Mortality is especially high among young individuals in resource-poor settings [28].

The greatest percentage of deaths from MALARIA occur in Nigeria, Democratic Republic of Congo, Burkina Faso, United Republic of Tanzania, Sierra-Leone, Niger and India. All of these countries, except India, had an increase in number of cases in 2017.

Of note, there is also geographic variation in *Plasmodium* species around the world. In Africa, Southeast Asia, Eastern Mediterranean regions, and Western Pacific regions, *Plasmodium falciparum* is the predominant species whereas in the Americas (where there were also significantly fewer cases), *Plasmodium vivax* is the predominant species. *Plasmodium falciparum* is known to cause more severe manifestations and is associated with higher mortality [29].

Diagnosis

Clinical Diagnosis

History can be somewhat helpful in the diagnosis of malaria. History should include questions regarding recent travel, especially to endemic regions. Early in the course of the illness, the disease severity and fever patterns can be unique based on the disease-causing organism.

Even for the experienced physician, the clinical diagnosis of malaria can be a difficult one to make due to the wide variation in presentation and nonspecific nature of the signs and symptoms.

Severe falciparum malaria is classified as having one of the following manifestations accompanied by *Plasmodium falciparum* parasitemia [30]:

- Impaired consciousness (Adults: GCS < 11)
- Generalized weakness
- More than two convulsions in a 24 hour period
- Acidosis
- Hypoglycemia (Adults: plasma glucose <40 mg/dL)
- Anemia (Adults: Hb $\leq$ 7 g/dL or Hct $\leq$ 20%) with 0.2% parasitemia
- Renal impairment (serum creatinine >3 mg/dL or blood urea >20 mmol/L)
- Jaundice (serum bilirubin >3 mg/dL) with 0.2% parasitemia
- Pulmonary edema confirmed by radiograph or O_2 saturation <92% on room air with respiratory rate >30/minute
- Prolonged or recurrent bleeding
- Shock
- Hyperparasitemia (>10% parasitemia)

Like many of the signs and symptoms of malaria, cutaneous manifestations can vary greatly and are relatively uncommon. There have been several case reports in which dermatologic manifestations accompanied the infection. There have been a few reported cases of patients presenting with urticaria and angioedema. Typically, these symptoms resolved and did not return upon treatment with antimalarials and antihistamines. Other morphologies that have been reported are a reticulated blotchy pattern, petechiae, and purpura. It is unclear why some patients present with mast cell mediated reactions and skin manifestations while others do not; most of these symptoms resolved with treatment of the underlying malaria [31]. There are also a few case reports of patients infected with malaria who demonstrated cutaneous manifestations of disseminated intravascular coagulation. Rare cases of purpura fulminans have been reported [32].

Laboratory Diagnosis

The gold standard for diagnostic testing for malaria is examination of peripheral blood (thick and thin smears) under a microscope. While there have been some other diagnostic tests used (rapid diagnostic tests detecting malaria antibodies, serological tests, etc.) these tests have varying degrees of sensitivity and specificity and are sometimes more expensive [33].

Treatment (Table 1)

Treatment is highly dependent on the disease severity, species of *Plasmodium*, and geographic region of likely source of infection [34].

Table 1

Severity	Species	Region	Treatment options
Uncomplicated malaria	*P. falciparum* or unidentified	Chloroquine-resistant	- Atovaquone-proguanil (Malarone™) - Artemether-lumefantrine (Coartem™) - Quinine sulfate + (doxycycline, tetracycline, or clindamycin) - Mefloquine (Lariam™)
		Chloroquine-sensitive	- Chloroquine phosphate (Aralen™) - Hydroxychloroquine (Plaquenil™)
	P. vivax or *P. ovale*	All regions (except chloroquine-resistant *P. vivax*)	- Chloroquine phosphate (Aralen™) + primaquine phosphate - Hydroxychloroquine (Plaquenil™) + primaquine phosphate
	P. vivax	Chloroquine-resistant	- Quinine sulfate + (doxycycline or tetracycline) + primaquine phosphate - Atovaquone-proguanil (Malarone™) + primaquine phosphate - Mefloquine + primaquine phosphate
Severe malaria (as defined under clinical diagnosis section)	N/A	All regions	- Quinidine gluconate + (doxycycline, tetracycline, or clindamycin)

Table 1 describes general treatment options for most adult populations; however, there are a few special patient groups to consider. Pregnant patients with uncomplicated malaria acquired from a chloroquine-sensitive region can receive chloroquine phosphate or hydroxychloroquine. Pregnant patients with uncomplicated malaria acquired from a chloroquine-resistant region can receive either mefloquine or quinine sulfate (plus clindamycin). Atovaquone-proguanil and artemether-lumefantrine are not recommended in pregnancy, especially during the first trimester. In pediatric patient groups, many of the same medications can be used as those described for the general adult population, with the exception of doxycycline and tetracycline in patients under the age of 8 [34].

Preventative measures

Bite avoidance and chemoprophylaxis for travelers

The two main tenets of malaria prevention are to prevent mosquito bites and to provide chemoprophylaxis to patients who are at risk for being bitten. Effective skin repellents include DEET 20–50% (applied every 6–12 hours), Picaridin 20% (applied every 6–12 hours), and lemon eucalyptus oil (requires more frequent application) [35].

Some ineffective repellents sometimes perceived to be useful by patients include homeopathic medications, yeast, garlic, marmite, vitamin B-1, electronic mosquito repellents, and citronella oil. The efficacy of these agents is not supported by the literature; therefore, they are not currently recommended [35].

Because of the wide variation in Plasmodium species globally, it is important to consider the region of travel and duration of travel before recommending chemoprophylaxis. Individual evaluation of risks and benefits made on a case-by-case basis has the potential to reduce the number of cases of travel- associated malaria (especially in high-risk individuals) while minimizing possible side effects of the medications in patients with other comorbidities. Chloroquine alone can be given in the case of travel to a region with chloroquine sensitivity. For individuals who are traveling to regions with limited chloroquine resistance, chloroquine plus proguanil can be given. For all other regions with widespread resistance, there are three main options for prophylaxis: atovaquone plus proguanil (Malarone™), doxycylcine, and mefloquine. While there is strong evidence to support malaria chemoprophylaxis, it is not effective in all cases. It is important to emphasize adherence to the regimen and educate patients about early signs and symptoms of the disease [35].

For high-risk travelers it is especially important to consider malaria prevention. Pregnant women should be encouraged to avoid travel to endemic areas when possible. Some options that are considered safe in pregnancy are DEET and the use of repellent nets. In terms of chemoprophylaxis, mefloquine and chloroquine can be used safely depending on resistance patterns in the region of travel. In children, the medication used is dependent upon the child's age and weight. Chloroquine plus proguanil can be used in all children, whereas mefloquine should be used in those weighing over 5 kg; doxycycline should only be used in children over the age of 8 [35].

Public Health Initiatives

Large scale public health initiatives have helped reduce the incidence of malaria in many countries. One research study explored interventions and their impact on malaria morbidity and mortality in Africa from 2000 to 2015 [36]. Insecticide-treated bednets had the greatest effect on reduction of disease (prevention of an estimated 68% of cases). The authors note that this may have had the greatest effect due to the ease of implementing this intervention early on a broader scale.

Culex

Classification of arthropod

Order Diptera, Suborder Nematocera, Family Culicidae, Genus Culex.

Description of arthropod

Culex mosquitoes have three sections (head, thorax, and abdomen). Several species from this genus are the main agents causing lymphatic filariasis, encephalitis virus and West Nile virus. These mosquitoes typically bite during the evening. Culex mosquitoes are laid as eggs in groups at the surface of water. A distinguishing characteristic of these mosquitoes is that their proboscis (nose) and body are at an angle to one another [37].

Clinical Diseases

Lymphatic Filiariasis

Transmission

There are a few disease causing nematode species, predominantly *Wuchereria bancrofti* but also *Brugia malayi* and *Brugia timori*. These worms are transmitted to humans via mosquitoes (*Culex*, *Anopheles*, *Aedes*, or *Mansonia*). Larvae deposit into the skin and subsequently enter lymphatics to mature into adult worms. In adult male patients, the adult worms are commonly found in the scrotal lymphatics, whereas in adult women and children, they are found in lymphatics along the upper and lower limbs. The adult worms cause dilation of the vessels, which over time leads to incompetence of the valves. The patient can eventually develop lymph stasis [38].

Epidemiology

Lymphatic filiariasis affects about 120 million people around the world and is mostly concentrated in tropical regions (Southeast Asia and Africa). Of these, 40 million have genital disease with a male predominance [39].

Diagnosis

Clinical manifestations include lymphedema and elephantiasis. This most commonly affects the lower limbs but can also affect the upper limbs and male genitalia.

Other skin changes can include hypertrichosis, hyperpigmentation, intertrigo in toe web spaces and chronic non-healing ulcers. Fungal infections are also common in advanced stages due to poor lymphatic flow. Although many patients are asymptomatic at early stages, these advanced findings can be debilitating [38].

Another manifestation is acute dermato-lymphangio-adenitis (ADLA) attacks believed to be precipitated by bacterial infections. These attacks are seen in higher areas of lymphedema and include pain, warmth, erythema, swelling and tenderness along with swollen and tender lymph nodes. Locally the attacks can lead to cellulitis or abscess formation and systemically, they cause fever, chills, headache and vomiting [38].

The diagnosis is usually made clinically since many tests (i.e. immune chromatographic test for filarial antigen detection and ultrasonography of the lymphatics) are commonly negative once lymphedema is established and patients are commonly asymptomatic at early stages [38].

Treatment

Diethylcarbemazine (DEC) is the treatment of choice for active infection; however, it only kills about half of adult worms and does not reverse the damage to lymphatics. Ivermectin and albendazole can also be used to reduce the number of worms. Severe ADLA attacks commonly require antibiotics such as penicillin, doxycycline, ampicillin, amoxicillin or cotrimoxazole. Although the specific bacteria is not commonly known, swabs of the entry site lesions can be cultured to help direct antibiotic therapy [38]. There has been strong evidence to suggest that a 6- week course of doxycycline is effective against *W. bancrofti* due to its strong macrofilaricidal activity and depletion of *Wolbachia* endosymbionts. Clinically, this resulted in a reduction of lymphatic vessel dilation and improvements in lymphedema [40].

Prevention

Primary prevention is of utmost importance, but there are several steps which can also prevent advancement of infection. Early treatment of the worms using DEC can prevent further damage to lymphatics. Foot hygiene and wound care can also be helpful in prevention of ADLA [38].

West Nile Virus

Transmission

West Nile Virus is caused by a flavivirus and is transmitted to humans mainly by the *Culex* mosquitoes globally. There have been case reports of *Aedes* mosquitoes also serving as vectors. Since humans do not have viral levels high enough to be transmitted back to mosquitoes, they are dead-end hosts. The incubation period lasts about 2–14 days, followed by onset of symptoms which can vary greatly (ranging from subclinical infection to encephalitis) [41].

Skin has been shown to play an important role in the transmission of disease from insects to humans. Mosquito saliva is injected into the dermis and contains some components which serve to liquefy the elastic dermal environment. Targeting those components to prevent viral entry into the dermal blood vessels has been an area of research interest [41].

Epidemiology

West Nile virus is relatively new to the Western Hemisphere. It was first diag-
nosed in individuals in New York during the summer of 1999. During the time
period from 2005 to 2009, there were almost 13,000 cases reported and of those
cases, about 35% had severe neurological manifestations (i.e. encephalitis).
Homelessness, cardiovascular disease, chronic kidney disease, hepatitis C infection, old age, and immunosuppression are risk factors for more severe disease and
death [41].

Diagnosis

Like many other infections, diagnosis is largely based on clinical manifestations
of the disease, which can be non-specific. While some patients are asymptomatic,
others may experience fever, myalgias and meningoencephalitis. In patients who
have encephalitis, progression can include flaccid paralysis of all four limbs.
Diagnosis can be confirmed by presence of IgM antibodies against the virus in the
cerebrospinal fluid [41].

Treatment

Currently, the only treatment option which exists is supportive care. There is no
FDA approved vaccine or specific treatment available, although it is the subject of
ongoing research.

Prevention

Application of insect repellents remains the mainstay of prevention. The general
guidelines for prevention of other mosquito-borne diseases, as outlined in detail
under the Malaria section, can be applied to West Nile virus.

Family Psychodidae

Phlebotomus

Classification of arthropod

Order Diptera, Suborder Nematocera, Family Psychodidae. Genus Phlebotomus.

Description of arthropod

Phlebotomine sandflies are typically small (less than 3.5 mm lengthwise) with
long legs. Color can vary between species (ranging from white to black) but can
be distinguished by a dense covering of hair and wings that appear to make a

V-shape at rest. They are most active at night and bites can go unnoticed by the host. Phlebotomine sandflies are most well-known for their transmission of old-world leishmaniasis [42].

Clinical Diseases

Old World Leishmaniasis

Transmission

Leishmaniasis is caused by a protozoan parasite transmitted to humans by sand-flies (from the genus *Phlebotomus*). In particular, the causative parasitic organisms for Old world cutaneous leishmaniasis are *L. major* (transmitted from animals), *L. tropica* (transmitted between humans), *L. aethiopica*, and *L. infantum*. Old world leishmaniasis is broadly distributed across the Middle East, Mediterranean, Arabian Peninsula, Africa and Asia [43].

Epidemiology

Phlebotomine sandflies are widely distributed around the world (Asia, Africa, Australia, southern Europe and the Americas). Clinical disease is common in the Mediterranean basin, central Asia and east Africa [42].

Diagnosis

There are varying degrees of involvement which leads to three forms of the disease: cutaneous leishmaniasis, mucocutaneous leishmaniasis, and visceral leishmaniasis. An erythematous papule first appears at the inoculation site which then enlarges, eventually forming a painless ulcer with a raised border. The ulcers can grow large, ranging from 0.5 cm to 10 cm in diameter. Although the lesions typically resolve over a period of 2–4 months, they leave a depressed scar [43].

Cutaneous manifestations can also vary based on the parasite species causing infection. For example, in *L. major* infection, there can be many ulcerated and crusted nodules. In *L. aethiopica*, there is a much slower progression of the ulceration which causes a more delayed healing process. *L. infantum* results in papules and nodules but minimal ulceration. In *L. tropica*, patients can develop leishmaniasis recidiva cutis [43].

In diffuse cutaneous leishmaniasis, the key difference is that the nodules do not ulcerate. This is most commonly seen in South and Central America [43].

There can be a wide range of presentations even beyond the predominant types discussed above. These can mimic many other dermatologic conditions such as lupus, psoriasis, and squamous cell carcinomas. Variations are especially common in immunosuppressed patients [43].

Since clinical diagnosis can be challenging, it has become important to correlate clinical and laboratory findings with patient history (living in or traveling to an endemic country). Options for laboratory diagnosis include smear, culture, PCR, histology and immunological tests [43].

Diagnostic method	Notes	Sensitivity	Specificity
Smear	Dermal smear from lesion margins using sterile surgical blade then bleached with May-Grunwald-Giemsa stain and observed under microscopy	64–80%	100%
Culture	Tissue fragment from active lesion margin incubated for 3–10 days at 28 °C in NNN/Schneider medium and observed under microscopy	40–84%	100%
PCR		98.8%	100%
Histology	4 mm punch biopsy from lesion margin; typical finding on H&E is a non-necrotizing granuloma; Giemsa stain can help identify the organisms with Leishman-Donovan bodies seen in macrophages or extracellularly	68%	–
Montenegro's reaction	Intradermal inoculation of 0.1 mL of Leishmania antigen in anterior forearm; considered positive if induration is >5 mm after 2–3 days	90%	–
Serological diagnosis	Indirect immunofluorescence and ELISA	Low	–

Treatment

There are several options for treatment of the disease. This is often directed based on the region of travel.

Medication	Mechanism of action	Side effects
Systemic treatments		
Pentavalent antimony derivatives (PAD)—Meglumine antimoniate, Stibogluconate	Unknown mechanism but possibly interferes with parasitic enzymes to prevent DNA synthesis	Fever, arthralgias/myalgias, GI upset, cardiotoxicity, pancreatitis, pancytopenia
Pentamidine	Prevents DNA synthesis of parasite	Hypertension, tachycardia, GI upset, rash
Metronidazole		
Amphotericin B		
Azoles		
Miltefosine	Oral antitumor agent	Hematological toxicity

Medication	Mechanism of action	Side effects
Allopurinol		
Doxycycline		
Azithromycin		
Rifampicine		
Oral zinc sulfates		
Local treatments		
Intralesional injection of PAD		
Paromomycin		
Imiquimod		
Thermotherapy		
CO_2 Laser		
Photodynamic therapy		
Electrotherapy		
Phytotherapy		

Prevention

Prevention of sand fly bites involves reducing exposure and wearing protective clothing, as outlined in detail under the Malaria section. The bites most commonly occur at night, so avoidance of outdoor activities at this time would be helpful. There is no effective vaccine against Leishmaniasis although significant efforts have been made to develop one. Part of the challenge has been that many tested vaccines are safe and immunogenic but do not result in effective long-term protection [44].

Sandfly Fever (Papatasi Fever)

Transmission

Sandfly fever is caused by a *Phlebovirus* transmitted to humans by *Phlebotomus* sandflies. The incubation period lasts from 3 to 6 days with symptoms typically lasting 3 days. The infection is sometimes referred to as "Three Day Fever" due to the duration of high fever (39–40 °C) [45].

Epidemiology

The disease is distributed primarily in the Mediterranean basin, northern parts of Africa, Middle East, and North India. There is variation among the causative viral species based on region, and this variation results in a range of clinical manifestations [46]. The predominant serotypes of *Phlebovirus* include Sand fly fever Sicilian virus (SFSV), Sand fly fever Naples virus (SFNV), and Toscana virus (TOSV). Infection is most common during the summer months because of increased activity of sandflies [45].

Diagnosis

Diagnosis is made clinically, but elevated IgM can be used for detection. Clinical manifestations are typically mild in most patients involving fever, other flu-like symptoms (headaches, myalgias, arthralgias, retro-orbital pain, chills) and GI discomfort. Laboratory findings include leukopenia, thrombocytopenia and elevations in AST and ALT. Severe forms present with acute encephalitis and are more commonly seen with the Toscana virus [45].

Skin manifestations observed in sandfly fever are usually related to an urticarial reaction. However, there have been two reported cases with patients experiencing a targetoid superficial erythematous skin lesion [45].

Treatment

The disease is treated symptomatically with fluids, rest, and analgesics. The disease is typically mild and associated with very low mortality [47].

Prevention

Since sandflies are susceptible to insecticides, it is possible to provide protection through use of treated bednets, curtains, clothes and sheets as well as repellents. Pyrethroid- treated bednets have been shown to result in a 50–65% reduction of disease.

Lutzomyia

Classification of arthropod

Order Diptera, Suborder Nematocera, Family Psychodidae, Genus Lutzomyia.

Description of arthropod

Lutzomyia sandflies are very similar to Phlebotomus sandflies (described above) but are more active near vegetation. They are well-known for their transmission of New World leishmaniasis [42].

Clinical Diseases

New World Leishmaniasis

Transmission

Leishmaniasis is caused by a protozoan parasite transmitted to humans by sandflies (from the genus *Lutzomyia*) [42]. In particular, the causative parasitic organisms for New World cutaneous leishmaniasis are *L. braziliensis, L. panamensis, L. peruviana, L. guyanensis, L. lainsoni, L. colombiensis, L. amazonensis, L. Mexicana, L. pifanoi, L. venezuelensis, and L. garnhami.* Additionally, *L. infanticum* is a species which can cause both Old and New world leishmaniasis [44].

Epidemiology

The geographical distribution of New World Leishmaniasis includes parts of South and Central America as well as Mexico. It is more commonly found near forested areas [42]. The *Lutzomyia* genus of sandflies is found in the region between the southern United States to northern Argentina. Most cases of cutaneous leishmaniasis occur in Brazil, Colombia and Peru [44]. Most cases of visceral leishmaniasis occur in Brazil [42].

Diagnosis

As the name suggests, cutaneous leishmaniasis begins with dermatological manifestations. There are two forms that are commonly seen: localized cutaneous leishmaniasis and disseminated cutaneous leishmaniasis. Initially in the localized form of disease, a small area of erythema appears at the site of the sandfly bite. This progresses into a papule, then nodule and eventually ulcerates. The time period during which the skin lesions progress from erythema to ulcer can vary from 2 weeks to 6 months. These lesions usually heal spontaneously but can result in significant scarring. Mucosal involvement has been observed in patients concurrently with the cutaneous manifestations, but has also been seen in patients 1–5 years after resolution of the initial cutaneous findings. The nasal mucosa is typically the first to be affected, resulting in inflammation, ulceration or septal perforation (known as espundia). This is much more difficult to treat than the cutaneous manifestations and can lead to mortality from secondary bacterial infections [44].

In the disseminated cutaneous form of the disease, there are non-ulcerative nodules which are dispersed on the entire body. This form is difficult to treat and does not usually resolve spontaneously.

While clinical presentation can assist with the diagnosis, the diagnosis can be confirmed with microscopic examination of Giemsa-stained smears, histopathological examination of biopsies or cultures or aspirates. Molecular parasitology can also be performed through PCR, but serology is rarely used to diagnose cutaneous leishmaniasis.

Clinical manifestations of visceral leishmaniasis include fever, hepatomegaly, splenomegaly, pancytopenia, anemia and weight loss. Skin involvement can also occur in the dermis. Although the gold standard for diagnosis is splenic biopsy to find parasites, this technique can be limited by the morbidity of the procedure. Thus, serological tests and molecular tests are often used. There is an immunochromatographic test for the rK39 antigen located in the kinesin region of the parasite. Diagnosis is typically made if this test is positive and the patient has had clinical symptoms (2 weeks of fever, splenomegaly and weight loss) [48].

Treatment

Treatment of cutaneous leishmaniasis is done in order to prevent scarring. Many endemic countries try to provide treatment for patients but with limited medication supply this can be difficult to accomplish. The recommended treatment for cutaneous leishmaniasis is with 20 mg/kg per day of sodium stibogluconate or meglumine antimonate for 20–28 days. These medications can have side effects including toxicity to the kidneys, liver, and heart. Amphotericin B can also be used in cases of mucosal involvement as well as in visceral leishmaniasis [44, 49].

Prevention

Prevention of New World Leishmaniasis is similar to that of Old World Leishmaniasis and is described under that section.

Family Simuliidae (Blackflies)

Simulium

Classification of arthropod

Order Diptera, Suborder Nematocera, Family Simuliidae, Genus Simulium.

Description of arthropod

Blackflies range in size from 5 mm to 15 mm and have an arched thorax. Most are black, but they can also have a yellow or orange body. They have large eyes and large wings and are best known for their transmission of onchocerciasis [50].

Clinical Diseases

Onchocerciasisis (River Blindness)

Transmission

Onchocerciasis is a parasitic disease caused by *Onchocerca volvulus,* transmitted via repeated blackfly bites. The flies typically live near rivers and streams and transfer *Onchocerca* larvae (microfilariae) through their bite to humans, where the parasites can reproduce. They mature over the next several months to a year and live in fibrous nodules in the skin (*onchocercomata*) to protect themselves from the human immune system. This allows the parasite to live in humans for several months to years. They produce more microfilariae which then can be taken up by blackflies and transmitted to other humans [51].

Epidemiology

Onchocercal infection is most common in sub-Saharan Africa but can also be found in parts of the Americas (Colombia, Ecuador, Mexico, Guatemala, Venezuela and Brazil) and in Yemen. At risk populations are individuals who live near rivers and streams where the blackflies live. Since many bites are typically needed in order to cause infection, it is less likely to occur in travelers to the area [52].

Diagnosis

Clinical manifestations can range from asymptomatic to severe. An increased number of bites typically correlates with an increased severity of infection, as they result in a larger burden of parasites within the human host. Onchocerciasis is a major cause of blindness worldwide. There are also several dermatological manifestations of this disease. Some patients can experience pruritic papular dermatitis while others develop lichenification of the skin. Patients can also have atrophy, depigmentation, and "peau-d'orange" secondary to edematous dermal change in the skin [53].

Definitive diagnosis can be made with skin snips containing adult worms in the excised nodules. This diagnostic method can have a low level of sensitivity, especially in cases of mild infection. While there are other methods of detection, some of them also depend on skin snips and there is no reliable technique for detection in resource-poor settings [53].

Treatment

Ivermectin is commonly used to treat onchocerciasis. Ivermectin obstructs the uterus of the worm to prevent microfilariae from being released. It can be given annually to patients over the age of five at a dose of 150 µg/kg body weight due to its low toxicity [53].

Prevention

Ivermectin is given annually to people at risk for the disease. It has greatly reduced the incidence of onchocerciasis and has prevented blindness in many patients [53].

Suborder Brachycera

Family Tabanidae

Tabanus

Classification of arthropod

Order Diptera, Suborder Brachycera, Family Tabanidae. Genus Tabanus.

Description of arthropod

Tabanus horse flies have bodies which consist of a head, thorax and abdomen. They measure 12.5–20.5 mm in length and are brown to black in color. The eyes are a distinguishing characteristic for these flies since they are brown/black but have a metallic green or red appearance in the light. Tabanid flies are primarily responsible for the transmission of loiasis. They are also capable of transmitting tularemia and anthrax, but are not the main vectors of transmission for these diseases [54].

Clinical Diseases

Loiasis

Transmission

Loiasis is caused by a filarial nematode (*Loa loa*) transmitted from human to human via tabanid flies. The main tabanid species which transmit loiasis in humans are *Chrysops silacea* and *C. dimidiata*. They bite most frequently in the mornings and late afternoons. The worms reside in the loose connective tissue under skin and produce microfilariae, which notably do not contain *Wolbachia* endosymbionts. These microfilariae can migrate through the bloodstream and can be found under the bulbar conjunctiva [55].

Epidemiology

Loiasis is most common in central Africa (Cameroon, Democratic Republic of the Congo, Gabon and Nigeria). It is important to note that the geographic distribution of loiasis is similar to that of onchocerciasis. In patients with high levels of *Loa Loa* worms in their bloodstream, there is a higher level of adverse events (fatal encephalopathy) if treatment for onchocerciasis with ivermectin is initiated. This creates a challenge in the treatment of onchocerciasis and has made the treatment in co-endemic areas the subject of research interest in the past several years [56].

Diagnosis

Clinical symptoms occur anywhere from a few months to decades after infection. Worm migration under the skin and in the eyes can be symptoms of this disease. Patients may also experience the appearance of Calabar swellings which are caused by hypersensitivity reactions to the parasite in the subcutaneous tissue. Symptoms can persist for years and include urticaria and pruritus.

Lab findings include eosinophilia, peripheral blood smear demonstrating microfilariae, and/or positive PCR detection of *Loa Loa*. Diagnosis can be made by removing the worm and observing it under a microscope [57].

Treatment

Treatment of loiasis is complicated because in patients with a high microfilariae levels, the antihelminthic effects can result in severe neurological side effects. Current recommendations are a 8–10 mg/kg/day dose of DEC for 21 days. Side effects to DEC (urticaria and Calabar swellings) can be treated with corticosteroids or antihistamines. Albendazole has also shown some activity against microfilariae [57].

Prevention

Prophylactic treatment with DEC 300 mg once a week can be administered to patients traveling to endemic areas. Otherwise, protective clothing and insect repellents (as described in the Malaria section) are the mainstay of prevention [58].

Family Muscidae

Tsetse

Classification of arthropod

Order Diptera, Suborder Brachycera, Family Muscidae. Genus Glossina.

Description of arthropod

Tsetse flies range in size from 8 mm to 17 mm and resemble house flies. They include all species in the genus *Glossina*. Distinguishing characteristics include a long proboscis and wings which fold directly on top of one another. There are about six species that are known to transmit parasites to humans and they are the primary vector for African sleeping sickness [59].

Clinical Diseases

Trypanosomiasis

Transmission

There are two main parasites responsible for transmission of sleeping sickness: *T.b. gambiense* and *T.b. rhodesiense*. The two forms are different in that *T.b. gambiense* is transmitted from human to human via the tsetse fly, whereas *T.b. rhodesiense* involves more transmission from domestic and wild animals to humans. Vertical transmission and transmission of disease through blood transfusion are also possible [60]. The parasite is initially in the blood stream and lymphatics but eventually gains access to the central nervous system through the CSF.

Epidemiology

The distribution of the two forms of disease also varies. *T.b. gambiense* is mostly found in central Africa, while *T.b. rhodesiense* is found in south and east Africa. Since 1995, the WHO has reported a decrease in new cases per year in Africa. from 300,000 to less than 10,000 new cases per year in 2009 [61].

Diagnosis

The *gambiense* form is chronic and can go undetected for months, whereas the *rhodesiense* form is acute and can result in death after a few months. In the *rhodesiense* form the initial skin manifestation is a furuncle which is present at the site of the tsetse fly bite.

After resolution, there is post-inflammatory hyperpigmentation that develops on the skin while the trypanosomes spread through the blood and lymph over a period of 2–3 weeks. After this period, the patient develops symptoms such as fever, headache, arthralgias, myalgias, rash (circular macules distributed across the trunk) and palpitations. If untreated, patients develop disturbances in sleep cycle, confusion, problems with coordination, coma and/or death. Patients with the *gambiense* form can develop the same symptoms, but it usually is more prolonged, presenting after about five years [62].

Diagnosis is made using laboratory methodology. Definitive diagnosis is made using microscopy of blood, lymph node fluid, or tissue biopsy (posterior cervical lymph node for *T.b. gambiense*) and observing parasites. Once they are identified, it is important to test the cerebrospinal fluid to determine the presence of neurological involvement. This will guide the choice of therapy for the patient. In these cases, CSF will demonstrate increased protein and a white cell count of greater than five [63].

Treatment

Treatment depends on stage of the infection. Early stage infection can be treated with pentamidine and suramin for either *T.b. gambiense* or *T.b. rhodesiense*. Eflornithine is used in second stage *T.b. gambiense* infection, either alone or in conjunction with nifurtimox. Melarsoprol is used for late stage *T.b. rhodesiense* and can also be used for late stage *T.b. gambiense* if needed [64].

Prevention

It is extremely difficult to prevent exposure to the tsetse fly in endemic areas; therefore, prevention efforts have focused on screening and preventing progression of the disease. Screening tools have been developed for at-risk populations in western and central Africa. The Card Agglutination Trypanosomiasis Test (CATT) is a serological screening that is only used for *T.b. gambiense* infections. It is important to detect disease early to prevent the devastating neurological effects that the disease can have if left untreated [64].

References

1. https://www.gatesnotes.com/Health/Most-Lethal-Animal-Mosquito-Week.
2. Centers for Disease Control. Dengue and the Aedes aegypti mosquito. 2012, January 30. Retrieved February 1, 2019, from https://www.cdc.gov/dengue/resources/30jan2012/aegyptifactsheet.pdf.
3. Centers for Disease Control. Comparison between main dengue vectors. 2012, January 30. Retrieved February 1, 2019, from https://www.cdc.gov/dengue/resources/30jan2012/comparisondenguevectors.pdf.
4. Centers for Disease Control. Dengue and the Aedes albopictus mosquito. 2012, January 30. Retrieved February 1, 2019, from https://www.cdc.gov/dengue/resources/30jan2012/albopictusfactsheet.pdf.
5. Higuera A, Ramírez JD. Molecular epidemiology of dengue, yellow fever, Zika and Chikungunya arboviruses: an update. Acta Trop. 2019;190:99–111. https://doi.org/10.1016/J.ACTATROPICA.2018.11.010.
6. Domingo C, Escadafal C, Rumer L, Mendez JA, Carcia P, Sall AA, …, Niedrig M. First international external quality assessment study on molecular and serological methods for yellow fever diagnosis. PLoS ONE. 2012;7(5):1–11. https://doi-org.ezproxy.libraries.wright.edu/10.1371/journal.pone.0036291.
7. Centers for Disease Control. Transmission of yellow fever virus. 2019, January 15. Retrieved March 3, 2019, from https://www.cdc.gov/yellowfever/transmission/index.html.
8. Lupi O, Tyring SK. Tropical dermatology: viral tropical diseases. J Am Acad Dermatol. 2003;49(6):979–1000. https://doi.org/10.1016/S0190-9622(03)02727-0.
9. Centers for Disease Control. Clinical and laboratory evaluation. 2015, August 21. Retrieved March 3, 2019, from https://www.cdc.gov/yellowfever/healthcareproviders/healthcareproviders-clinlabeval.html.
10. Sako EY, Rubin A, Young LC. Localized bullous fixed drug eruption following yellow fever vaccine. J Am Acad Dermatol. 2014;70:e113–4.
11. Karouni M, Kurban M, Abbas O. Lichen striatus following yellow fever vaccination in an adult woman. Clin Exp Dermatol. 2017;42(7):823–4. https://doi.org/10.1111/ced.13167.
12. Julander JG. Experimental therapies for yellow fever. Antiviral Res. 2012;97(2):169–79.
13. Centers for Disease Control. Yellow fever vaccine recommendations. 2019, January 16. Retrieved March 3, 2019, from https://www.cdc.gov/yellowfever/vaccine/vaccine-recommendations.html.
14. World Health Organization. Dengue and severe dengue. 2018, September 13. Retrieved March 5, 2019, from https://www.who.int/news-room/fact-sheets/detail/dengue-and-severe-dengue.
15. Thomas EA, John M, Kanish B. Mucocutaneous manifestations of dengue fever. Indian J Dermatol. 2010;55(1):79–85.
16. Rajapakse S, Rodrigo C, Rajapakse AC. Treatment of dengue fever. Infect Drug Resist. 2012;5:103–12.
17. World Health Organization. Chikungunya. 2012, April 26. Retrieved from https://www.who.int/ith/diseases/chikungunya/en/.
18. Centers for Disease Control. Chikungunya virus in the United States | Chikungunya virus | CDC. n.d. Retrieved February 1, 2019, from https://www.cdc.gov/chikungunya/geo/united-states.html.

19. Inamadar AC, Palit A, Sampagavi VV, Raghunath S, Deshmukh NS. Cutaneous manifestations of chikungunya fever: observations made during a recent outbreak in south India. Int J Dermatol. 2008;47(2):154–9. https://doi.org/10.1111/j.1365-4632.2008.03478.x.
20. LaRocque RL, Ryan ET. Personal actions to minimize mosquito-borne illnesses, including Zika virus. Ann Intern Med;165:589–590. https://doi.org/10.7326/m16-1397.
21. Farahnik B, Beroukhim K, Blattner CM, Young J. Cutaneous manifestations of the Zika virus. J Am Acad Dermatol. 2016;74(6):1286–7. https://doi.org/10.1016/J.JAAD.2016.02.1232.
22. Centers for Disease Control. Transmission methods. 2019, January 9. Retrieved February 5, 2019, from https://www.cdc.gov/zika/prevention/transmission-methods.html.
23. MacDonald PDM, Holden EW. Zika and public health: understanding the epidemiology and information environment. Pediatrics. 2018;141(2):S137–45. https://doi.org/10.1542/peds.2017-2038B.
24. Satterfield-Nash A, Kotzky K, Allen J, et al. Health and development at age 19–24 months of 19 children who were born with microcephaly and laboratory evidence of congenital Zika virus infection during the 2015 Zika virus outbreak. MMWR Morb Mortal Wkly Rep. 2017;66:1347–52. doi:http://dx.doi.org/10.15585/mmwr.mm6649a2.
25. Wolford RW, Schaefer TJ. Zika virus. [Updated 2018 Nov 14]. In: StatPearls [Internet]. Treasure Island (FL): StatPearls Publishing; 2019 January. https://www.ncbi.nlm.nih.gov/books/NBK430981/.
26. Rawal G, Yadav S, Kumar R. Zika virus: an overview. J Fam Med Prim Care. 2016;5(3):523–7. https://doi.org/10.4103/2249-4863.197256.
27. Malaria. 2018, November 14. Retrieved February 1, 2019, from https://www.cdc.gov/malaria/about/biology/index.html.
28. Centers for Disease Control. Malaria's impact worldwide. n.d. Retrieved February 1, 2019, from https://www.cdc.gov/malaria/malaria_worldwide/impact.html.
29. World Health Organization. World Malaria Report 2018. Geneva; 2018. License: CC BY-NC-SA 3.0 IGO.
30. World Health Organization. Guidelines for the treatment of malaria, 3rd ed. Geneva; 2015.
31. Vaishnani JB. Cutaneous findings in five cases of malaria. Indian J Dermatol Venereol Leprol. 2011;77(1):110. Retrieved February 5, 2019, from http://www.ijdvl.com/article.asp?issn=0378-6323;year=2011;volume=77;issue=1;spage=110;epage=110;aulast=Vaishnani.
32. Sharma A, Sharma V. Purpura fulminans: an unusual complication of malaria. Braz J Infect Dis. 2013;17(6):712–3. https://doi.org/10.1016/j.bjid.2013.04.013.
33. Tangpukdee N, Duangdee C, Wilairatana P, Krudsood S. Malaria diagnosis: a brief review. Korean J Parasitol. 2009;47(2):93–102.
34. Centers for Disease Control. Guidelines for treatment of malaria in the United States. 2013, July 1. Retrieved February 1, 2019, from https://www.cdc.gov/malaria/resources/pdf/treatmenttable.pdf.
35. Lalloo DG, Hill DR. Preventing malaria in travellers. BMJ (Clin Res Ed). 2008; 336(7657):1362–6
36. Bhatt S, Weiss DJ, Cameron E, Bisanzio D, Mappin B, Dalrymple U, Battle K, Moyes CL, Henry A, Eckhoff PA, Wenger EA, Briët O, Penny MA, Smith TA, Bennett A, Yukich J, Eisele TP, Griffin JT, Fergus CA, Lynch M, Lindgren F, Cohen JM, Murray C, Smith DL, Hay SI, Cibulskis RE, … Gething PW. The effect of malaria control on Plasmodium falciparum in Africa between 2000 and 2015. Nature. 2015;526(7572):207–11.
37. World Health Organization. Mosquitoes and other biting diptera. Retrieved April 7, 2019, from https://www.who.int/water_sanitation_health/resources/vector007to28.pdf.
38. Shenoy RK. Clinical and pathological aspects of filarial lymphedema and its management. Korean J Parasitol. 2008;46(3):119–25. https://doi.org/10.3347/kjp.2008.46.3.119.
39. World Health Organization. Lymphatic filariasis epidemiology. Retrieved April 5, 2019, from https://www.who.int/lymphatic_filariasis/epidemiology/en/.

40. Debrah AY, Mand S, Specht S, Marfo-Debrekyei Y, Batsa L, Pfarr K, …, Hoerauf A. Doxycycline reduces plasma VEGF-C/sVEGFR-3 and improves pathology in lymphatic filariasis. PLoS Pathog. 2006;2(9):e92. https://doi.org/10.1371/journal.ppat.0020092.
41. Colpitts TM, Conway MJ, Montgomery RR, Fikrig E. West Nile virus: biology, transmission, and human infection. Clin Microbiol Rev. 2012;25(4):635–48. https://doi.org/10.1128/cmr.00045-12.
42. Maroli M, Feliciangeli D, Bichaud L, Charrel R, Gradoni L. Phlebotomine sandflies and the spreading of leishmaniases and other diseases of public health concern. Medical Vet Entomol J. 2012;27:123–47.
43. Masmoudi A, Hariz W, Marrekchi S, Amouri M, Turki H. Old world cutaneous leishmaniasis: diagnosis and treatment. J Dermatol Case Rep. 2013;7(2):31–41. https://doi.org/10.3315/jdcr.2013.1135.
44. Reithinger R, Dujardin JC, Louzir H, Pirmez C, Alexander B, Brooker S. Cutaneous leishmaniasis. Lancet Infect Dis. 2007;7:581–96.
45. Temocin F, Sari T, Tulek N. Sandfly fever with skin lesions: a case series from Turkey. J Arthropod-Borne Dis. 2016;10(4):608–12.
46. Kocak Tufan Z, Tasyaran MA, Guven T. Sandfly fever: a mini review. Virol Mycol. 2013;2:109.
47. Özkale Y, Özkale M, Kiper P, Çetinkaya B, Erol İ. Sadfly fever: two case reports. Turk Pediatr Ars. 2016;51(2):110–3. https://doi.org/10.5152/TurkPediatriArs.2015.1734.
48. Sundar S. Visceral leishmaniasis. Trop Parasitol. 2015;5(2), 83–85. https://doi.org/10.4103/2229-5070.162487.
49. Moore EM, Lockwood DN. Treatment of visceral leishmaniasis. J Glob Infect Dis. 2010;2(2):151–8. https://doi.org/10.4103/0974-777X.62883.
50. Hill CA, Platt J, MacDonald JF. Black flies: biology and public health risk. 2010, May. Retrieved April 30, 2019, from https://extension.entm.purdue.edu/publications/E-251.pdf.
51. Centers for Disease Control. Onchocerciasis disease. 2013, May 21. Retrieved April 29, 2019, from https://www.cdc.gov/parasites/onchocerciasis/disease.html.
52. Centers for Disease Control. Onchocerciasis epidemiology and risk factors. 2013, May 21. Retrieved April 29, 2019, from https://www.cdc.gov/parasites/onchocerciasis/epi.html.
53. Stingl P. Onchocerciasis: developments in diagnosis, treatment and control. Int J Dermatol. 2009;48(4):393–6. https://doi.org/10.1111/J.1365-4632.2009.03843.X.
54. Desquesnes M, Wongthangsiri D, Jittapalapong S, Chareonviriyaphap T. Guidelines for user-friendly iconographic description of hematophagous flies' external morphology; application to the identification of Tabanus rubidus (Wiedemann, 1821) (Diptera: Tabanidae). J Asia-Pac Entomol. 2018;21(3):807–22. https://doi.org/10.1016/J.ASPEN.2018.06.005.
55. Whittaker C, Walker M, Pion SD, Chesnais CB, Boussinesq M, Basáñez M. The population biology and transmission dynamics of loa loa. Trends Parasitol. 2018;34(4):335–50. https://doi.org/10.1016/J.PT.2017.12.003.
56. Whittaker C, Walker M, Pion SD, Chesnais CB, Boussinesq M, Basáñez M. The population biology and transmission dynamics of loa loa. Trends in Parasitology. 2018;34(4):335–50. https://doi.org/10.1016/j.pt.2017.12.003.
57. Sadia A, Fisher M, Juckett G. The African eye worm: a case report and review. J Travel Med. 2008;15(1):50–2. https://doi.org/10.1111/j.1708-8305.2007.00166.x.
58. Centers for Disease Control. Loiasis prevention and control. 2015, Jan 20. Retrieved April 30, 2019, from https://www.cdc.gov/parasites/loiasis/prevent.html.
59. World Health Organization. Human African Trypansomiasis the vector (tsetse fly). Retrieved April 30, 2019, from https://www.who.int/trypanosomiasis_african/disease/vector/en/.
60. World Health Organization. Human African Trypansomiasis the transmission cycle. Retrieved April 30, 2019, from https://www.who.int/trypanosomiasis_african/disease/transmission_cycle/en/.

61. World Health Organization. Human African Trypansomiasis epidemiological situation. Retrieved April 30, 2019, from https://www.who.int/trypanosomiasis_african/country/en/.

62. Natuva DP, Brahmani S, Subbarao K, Padma B, Anil B, Koppulo S, Rao CB. Molecular mechanisms and therapeutic approaches to the treatment of African Trypanosomiasis. Drug Inven Today. 2012;4(5):381–388. Retrieved from https://search-ebscohost-com.ezproxy. libraries.wright.edu/login.aspx?direct=true&db=a9h&AN=100835130&site=eds-live.

63. Centers for Disease Control. Sleeping sickness diagnosis. 2012, Aug 29. Retrieved April 30, 2019, from https://www.cdc.gov/parasites/sleepingsickness/diagnosis.html.

64. World Health Organization. Human African Trypansomiasis symptoms, diagnosis and treatment. Retrieved April 30, 2019, from https://www.who.int/trypanosomiasis_african/disease/ diagnosis/en/.

Millipede

Neda Shahriari, Mohammed Malik and Brett Sloan

Introduction

The millipede is one of the oldest recorded terrestrial organisms [1]. With approximately 12,000 species currently named, millipedes make up the scientific class *Diplopoda*. The size and shape of a millipede is quite variable ranging from 2 mm to almost 40 cm [2]. The major dermatologic condition from millipede exposure is contact dermatitis resulting in a mahogany–colored burn, most often on the hands/forearms and feet [3].

Classification and Epidemiology

Millipedes comprise the scientific class *Diplopoda*, derived from Ancient Greek words for "double foot" [1]. Indeed, it is the two pairs of legs on most body segments that distinguish the millipede from other arthropods within the subphylum Myriapoda, such as centipedes, which have just one pair of legs per body segment. Millipedes and centipedes can be further distinguished through their diets—the majority of millipedes are detritivores while centipedes are carnivores [2].

Within the *Diplopoda* class, there are three major subclasses that make up the 12,000 identified millipede species [4]. The subclass Penicillata contains only one living order—Polyxenida. The Polyxenida order (of which there are currently 86 species) can be distinguished by their soft, non-calcified exoskeleton, as well as the abundance of bristles on their body, thus coining the term

N. Shahriari (✉) · M. Malik · B. Sloan
Department of Dermatology, University of Connecticut Health Center, 21 South Road, Farmington, CT 06032, USA
e-mail: shahriari@uchc.edu

B. Sloan
e-mail: Steven.Sloan@va.gov

© Springer Nature Switzerland AG 2020
J. Trevino and A. Y-Y. Chen (eds.), *Dermatological Manual of Outdoor Hazards*,
https://doi.org/10.1007/978-3-030-37782-3_12

"bristled millipedes". The subclass Arthropleuridea is extinct. The final subclass, Chilognatha, contains the remaining living millipede species. The classification of millipedes is incomplete—it is suspected that there are thousands more species left to discover, and the position of the orders within *Diplopoda* is not entirely agreed upon [4].

Millipedes are generally considered harmless to humans [2]. Only their secretions can cause dermatologic conditions. However, they can be an agricultural or household pest. *Xenobolus carnifex* is known to infest thatched roofs in South India and Sri Lanka [5], while *Ommatoiulus moreleti* invades homes in Australia during the autumn months [6]. *Blaniulus guttulatus* infests sugar beets and root crops and is found across Europe and North America [7]. On the other hand, millipedes have been used in traditional medicine worldwide to help heal a variety of ailments [8, 9].

Anatomy and Physiology

Millipedes are cylindrical arthropods consisting of a head with antennae and trunk [1]. The first segment of the trunk is known as the collum and does not contain any legs. The majority of the body rings composing the trunk consist of two pairs of legs per segment (diplosegment), with the exception of the first three rings that contain only one leg per segment and the last few which are legless [1, 2]. This anatomy allows for robust burrowing. The seventh body ring determines the sex of the millipede, with males containing *gonopods,* which are sperm transfer organs, instead of legs [2]. The exoskeleton of the millipede is calcified and consists of three layers including epicuticle, exocuticle and endocuticle [2].

Millipedes have a sophisticated chemical defense system designed to ward off potential harm. With the exception of a few specific millipede orders, all others have repugnatorial glands for production of noxious chemicals, which are extruded from pores along the millipede's sides [1, 10–12]. The chemical composition of millipede secretions includes p-benzoquinones, p-cresol, phenol, quinazolinones, alkaloids, terpenoids, and cyanogenic glycosides [1].

Clinical Disease

Although uncommon, the clinical manifestations of millipede exposure are related to the release of the noxious chemicals in its defense system armamentarium. Upon exposure to the skin, these chemicals result in an irritant contact dermatitis causing a burn-like reaction of the skin with dyspigmentation [13, 14]. Exposure of the eye to the chemicals is quite serious, causing pain and inflammation with subsequent risk for corneal ulceration and blindness [13, 14]. Common areas of exposure include the hands and forearms, since children are more likely to pick up millipedes [15].

Furthermore, since millipedes may hide in shoes, contact here leads to lesions on the feet (Fig. 1) [3, 15, 16]. The dyspigmentation typically seen with millipede exposure is thought to be due to a combination of quinone oxidation, yielding a mahogany discoloration, and the presence of hydroquinone in the chemical defense system resulting in areas of depigmentation [15]. In addition to cutaneous pigmentation following exposure, individuals often experience a localized burning sensation. If contact time is increased, blistering and ulceration may occur [17].

Diagnosis

Knowledge of exposure to a millipede leaves little diagnostic doubt when facing cutaneous discoloration resembling a superficial burn. However, lack of exposure history does pose a challenge for the clinician. The lesion needs to be distinguished from burns related to hot objects; however, the mahogany discoloration is characteristic of millipede burns [15]. Further, the area may resemble bruises with the noted variegate coloration that occurs in the natural healing process. Child abuse needs to be carefully teased out given millipede burns are more common

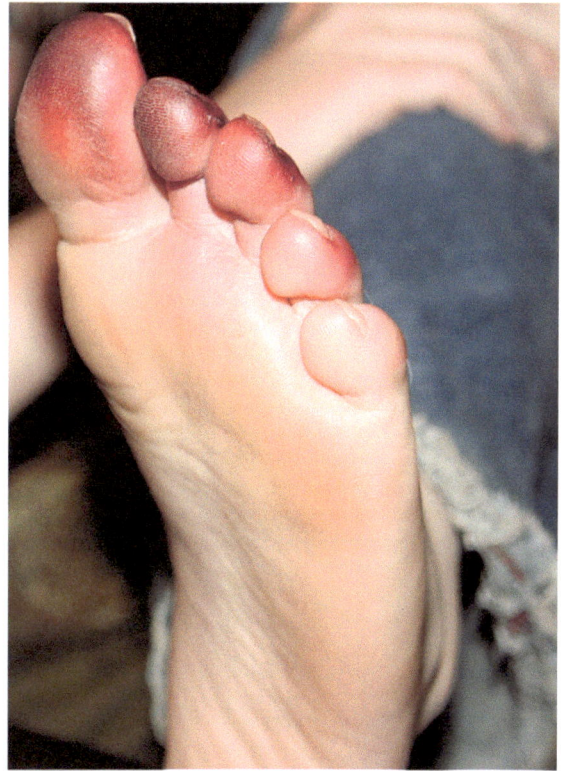

Fig. 1 Irritant contact dermatitis following millipede toxin exposure. This reaction followed child putting on her shoe and crushing the millipede. Attribution: User Tmera—English-language Wikipedia, Public Domain https://commons.wikimedia.org/w/index.php?curid=1914101

Table 1 Sample cases of millipede burns in the literature

Cutaneous symptoms	Other symptoms	Route of exposure	Differential diagnosis	Treatment	Outcome	Source
Cyanotic and erythematous macules on the first three toes of the right foot	Local pain and paresthesia	Stepped on "millipede"	Ischemic cyanosis	Analgesia and observation	Inflammation subsided, pigmentation remained for months	Lima et al. [18]
Brownish-red discoloration of the vulvar region with small amount of desquamation and linear fissure	Mild mucopurulent discharge. Tenderness in area	Dead elongated insect noted in the child's clothing	Child abuse	Oral amoxicillin/potassium clavulanate and local application of topical steroid and antibacterial agents	Healing of fissure and reduction of swelling and erythema. There was formation of mahogany-colored crust over clitoral region. With healing, depigmentation of surrounding area noted. Discharge from hospital after 6 days	Dar et al. [15]
Mild hyperemia of the oral mucosa	None	Millipede found in between the lips	NA	None	Complete resolution	De Capitani et al. [17]
Toes initially appeared yellow, transitioned to brown color after an hour	Burning sensation immediately after exposure	Millipede in shoe	NA	Cleansed with soap and water	NA	Hendrickson [3]

NA = Not Available

amongst the younger population [15]. At times, the discoloration has resembled ischemic tissue due to the dark reddish or blackish staining [18]. Table 1 summarizes a few cases reported in the literature with unique features to highlight differential diagnosis and diagnostic dilemmas. The ability of the clinician to accurately identify a patient's cutaneous reaction as a manifestation of millipede exposure has profound consequences including curbing unnecessary procedures and saving health care dollars.

Treatment

Management of cutaneous millipede burns requires thorough washing with soap and water to dilute the toxic substances. Otherwise, care is mainly supportive including analgesics, topical corticosteroids depending on the severity of presentation, and medical reassurance [17]. The use of topical ethyl ether solution, which contains benzoquinone solvent properties, has been suggested by some individuals; however, no efficacy data is available [17, 19]. Resolution of pigmentation takes several weeks to months [20]. Preventive measures include shaking shoes and turning socks inside out to avoid accidental exposures [17].

References

1. Sierwald P, Bond JE. Current status of the myriapod class Diplopoda (millipedes): taxonomic diversity and phylogeny. Annu Rev Entomol. 2007;52:401–20.
2. Lewbart GA, editor. Invertebrate medicine. Wiley; 2011.
3. Hendrickson RG. Millipede exposure. Clin Toxicol. 2005;43(3):211–2.
4. Shear WA, Edgecombe GD. The geological record and phylogeny of the Myriapoda. Arthropod Struct Dev. 2010;39(2–3):174–90.
5. Alagesan PE, Muthukrishnan JA. Bioenergetics of the household millipede pest, Xenobolus carnifex (Fabricius, 1775) (Diplopoda: Spirobolida). Peckiana. 2005;4:3–14.
6. McKillup SC. Behaviour of the millipedes Ommatoiulus moreletii, Ophyiulus verruculiger and Oncocladosoma castaneum in response to visible light; an explanation for the invasion of houses by Ommatoiulus moreletii. J Zool. 1988;215(1):35–46.
7. Blower JG. Millipedes: keys and notes for the identification of the species. Brill Archive; 1985.
8. Lawal OA, Banjo AD. Survey for the usage of arthropods in traditional medicine in southwestern Nigeria. J Entomol. 2007;4(2):104–12.
9. Negi CS, Palyal VS. Traditional uses of animal and animal products in medicine and rituals by the Shoka Tribes of District Pithoragarh, Uttaranchal, India. Ethno-Med. 2007;1(1):47–54.
10. Arab A, Zacarin GG, Fontanetti CS, Camargo-Mathias MI, dos Santos MG, Cabrera AC. Composition of the defensive secretion of the Neotropical millipede Rhinocricus padergi Verhoeff 1938 (Diplopoda: Spirobolida: Rhinocricidae). Entomotropica. 2003;18:79–82.
11. Eisner T, Alsop D, Hicks K, Meinwald J. Defensive secretions of millipedes. In: Bettini S, editor. Arthropod venoms. Berlin: Springer; 1978. pp. 41–72.

12. Burns DA. Diseases caused by arthropods and other noxious animals. In: Burns T, Breathnach SM, Cox N, Griffiths C, editors. Rook/Wilkinson/Ebling textbook of dermatology, vol 3. Oxford, UK: Blackwell Science; 2004. pp. 33.55–33.56.

13. Hudson BJ, Parsons GA. Giant millipede 'burns' and the eye. Trans R Soc Trop Med Hyg. 1997;91:183–5.

14. Pollack, RJ, Norton SA. Ectoparasite infestations and arthropod injuries. In: Larry Jameson J, et al editors. Harrison's principles of internal medicine, 20e. New York: McGraw-Hill; 2015. http://accessmedicine.mhmedical.com/content.aspx?bookid=2129&sectionid=192534409. Accessed 10 Apr 2019.

15. Dar NR, Raza N, Rehman SB. Millipede burn at an unusual site mimicking child abuse in an 8-year-old girl. Clin Pediatr. 2008;47(5):490–2.

16. Elston DM. What's eating you? millipede (Diplopoda). Cutis. 2001;67:452.

17. De Capitani EM, Vieira RJ, Bucaretchi F, Fernandes LC, Toledo AS, Camargo AC. Human accidents involving Rhinocricus spp., a common millipede genus observed in urban areas of Brazil. Clin Toxicol. 2011;49(3):187–90.

18. Lima CA, Cardoso JL, Magela A, de Oliveira FG, Talhari S, Haddad Junior V. Exogenous pigmentation in toes feigning ischemia of the extremities: a diagnostic challenge brought by arthropods of the Diplopoda Class ("millipedes"). Anais brasileiros de dermatologia. 2010;85(3):391–2.

19. Haddad V Jr, Cardoso JLC. Accidents provoked by millipede with dermatological manifestations: report of two cases. An Bras Dermatol. 2000;75:471–4.

20. Verma AK, Bourke B. Millipede burn masquerading as trash foot in a paediatric *patient*. ANZ J Surg. 2014;84(5):388–90.

Centipedes

Neda Shahriari and Brett Sloan

Introduction

Centipedes are flattened arthropods that are infrequently the cause of cutaneous reactions. The non-specific nature of the eruption resulting from centipede exposure often makes it difficult to ascertain the accurate etiologic agent. An understanding of centipede classification, epidemiology, and anatomy and physiology is crucial to guide clinicians in the proper diagnosis and management of pertinent clinical manifestations.

Classification and Epidemiology

The word centipede is derived from the Latin prefix *centi-* for "hundred" and *pedis* "foot", although different species vary in the total number of legs. Centipedes are invertebrates classified as a component of the Arthropoda phylum and Myriapoda subphylum [1]. Amongst the myriapods, centipedes are a constituent of the Chilopoda class with over 3000 species of centipedes catalogued into five orders: Geophilomorpha ("earth centipedes"), Scolopendromorpha (giant centipedes Fig. 1), Lithobiomorpha ("stone centipedes"), Craterostigmomorpha, and Scutigeromorpha ("house centipedes") [1]. The unifying feature for the Chilopoda class is the modified first pair of appendages known as forcipules, which is utilized to capture prey and inject venom [2].

N. Shahriari (✉) · B. Sloan
Department of Dermatology, University of Connecticut Health Center,
21 South Road, Farmington, CT 06032, USA
e-mail: shahriari@uchc.edu

B. Sloan
e-mail: Steven.Sloan@va.gov

© Springer Nature Switzerland AG 2020
J. Trevino and A. Y-Y. Chen (eds.), *Dermatological Manual of Outdoor Hazards*,
https://doi.org/10.1007/978-3-030-37782-3_13

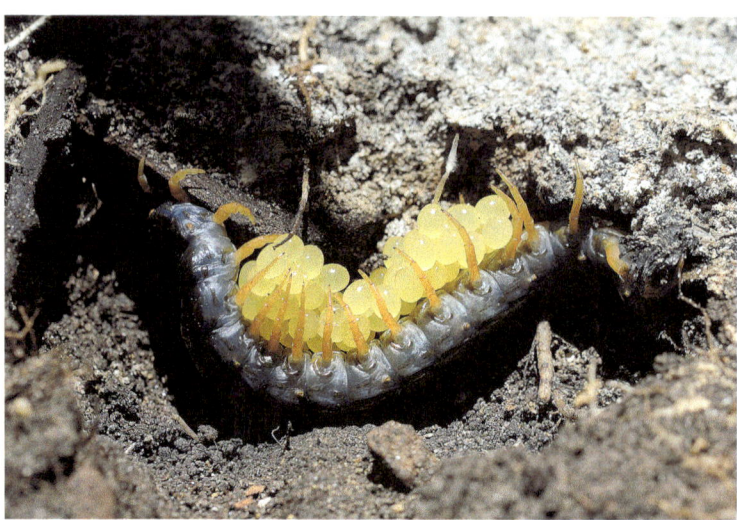

Fig. 1 Centipede, *Cormocephalus aurantiipes,* Scolopendridae family, Scolopendromorpha order. By Chicquita Burke [Public domain] https://commons.wikimedia.org/wiki/File:Orange-footed_centipede.jpg

The estimated number of Chilopoda species in the world is between 6,850–6,950 with over 3,196 of which have been officially documented and described [3]. Centipedes are found worldwide and are attracted to moist and dark environments including beneath rocks, rotting wood, moist basements, and moist soils. Centipedes are highly attracted to tropical environments since these regions are warm and humid [4]. Since centipedes are terrestrial creatures, they are not found in aquatic environments, though they will occasionally inhabit regions along the water's edge to seek the benefits of moisture. The aforementioned is characteristic of the Geophilomorpha order. Though counterintuitive given the arid environment, centipedes in the order Scolopendromorpha can be found in deserts where they avoid the sun by seeking shelter in shade and disappearing into crevices [4]. Centipedes may be found in moist, dark areas of houses. They are not only attracted to houses by virtue of environmental factors, but also the potential to access preferred food sources including small insects and spiders. An understanding of suitable habitats that attract centipedes is significant for clinicians in ascertaining the likelihood of a cutaneous reaction due to centipede exposure.

Anatomy and Physiology

Given the different orders of centipedes, it should come as no surprise that the centipedes harbor varying features amongst their cohort. Their length can range from just a few millimeters to as large as 30 cm as observed in *Scolopendra gigantean* [4]. The centipede anatomy is simply composed of a head and trunk. The trunk is composed of multiple segments, ranging from 15 to 191, with the first segment containing the forcipules or poison claws [5]. Each forcipule contains poisonous glands utilized by centipedes on their prey. Each of the remaining segments on the trunk contains a pair of legs. Centipedes have a posterior genital opening (opisthogoneate) used for reproduction [4].

The anatomic relevance of centipedes in the human-centipede interaction comes from the venomous secretions of the forcipules. Forcipules are shaped like forceps and each is composed of four different segments [6]. At the tip of the claw, there is a pore for secretion of venom, which is directly connected to venom gland via a chitinous venom duct [6]. There is a myriad of bioactive proteins comprising the centipede's venom. This includes phospholipase A2, metalloproteinases, acid and alkaline phosphatases, and esterases, which comprise the enzymatic proteins [7]. The components of non-enzymatic proteins include neurotoxic, myotoxic, hemolytic, and cardiotoxic substances [7].

The exoskeleton of a centipede lacks the waxy layer observed in the other Arthropoda phylum and therefore moisture retention is problematic [8]. It is for this reason Centipedes are attracted to moist environments in order to prevent dehydration.

Clinical Disease

Though centipede stings occur frequently, they often don't come to medical attention since most are fairly mild and afflicted individuals do not report to physicians. Fatalities associated with centipede stings have typically not been associated with the actual venom but rather secondary infection at the site of centipede sting [9].

Centipedes have a predilection for biting on the hands and feet at night [10–12]. Classically, centipede bites leave two puncture wounds at the site of fang penetration and result in erythema and edema of the surrounding area [9–14]. Other cutaneous manifestations of centipede bites include hemorrhagic vesicles, blisters, pustules and necrosis [11]. There can be associated numbness and paresthesia at affected site, lymphangitis and bacterial superinfection [9, 11, 15]. Pain associated with centipede bite may be significant in nature. Pruritus and burning are other sensations that may be experienced locally as well. Table 1 depicts sample cases within the literature to demonstrate different manifestations and sequela of centipede bites and exposure.

The most common systemic manifestations of centipede envenomation include headache, dizziness, lethargy, and nausea. Rare cases of anaphylaxis have been reported in the literature [16–18; Table 1]. Furthermore, rhabdomyolysis [19], myocardial ischemia [20], and Well's syndrome [21] have rarely been reported (see Table 1).

The components of centipede venom result in the clinical manifestations delineated above. Centipede envenomation leads to the release of histamine and serotonin neurotransmitters in the host, yielding localized neurologic symptoms [7].

Table 1 Sample cases depicting various manifestations of centipede bites and exposures

Subspecies	Cutaneous Symptoms	Other symptoms	Other findings	Treatment	Outcome	Source
S. subspinipes	Erythematous edema, round in shape, bright red in color with diameter of 5 cm	Acute pain	Leukocytosis (11,300) and increased ESR (first hour 51 mm)	Paracematol (2 g/day) and oral prednisone (starting daily dose of 50 mg)	Improvement within 5 days, complete remission in two weeks	Veraldi et al.
S. subspinipes	1.5 cm bulla, containing clear serous fluid, surrounded by erythematous halo	Severe burning and pain	Leukocytosis (12,600) and ESR (first hour 59 mm)	Paracematol (2 g/day) and oral prednisone (starting daily dose of 50 mg)	Improvement within 5 days, complete remission in two weeks	Veraldi et al.
S. subspinipes	Edema of left hand at site of centipede bite	Anaphylaxis		Adrenaline	Improvement after 1 day	Washio et al.
Scolopendra	Edema of lower leg at the site of centipede bite which progressed to ulceration	Dizziness, chills. With time, eventual weakness and weight loss	Wound smears showed non-toxigenic strains of *C. diphtheriae*	Erythromycin 1000 mg given 4 times daily IV, chinosol dressing	Improvement after 10 days of treatment	Jungling et al.
S. subspinipes (Patient ingested alcohol soaked with centipede)	Erythematous swelling of the bilateral upper extremities and trunk with bullae	Neurologic deficits: right wrist drop, impaired left hand grasp, paresthetic sensation of bilateral hands	Leukocytosis of 21,500 with left shift. Creatinine 2.0, myoglobin 23,543 consistent with rhabdomyolysis	IV isotonic saline. Hydrocortisone 100 mg IV every 8 hours for 1 week	Improvement in labs on the 9th day of hospitalization. Neurologic deficits remained requiring outpatient rehabilitation	Wang et al.
Likely Scutigera coleoptrata	Edema, bullae and pruritus of bilateral hands, which two weeks later progressed to violaceous, indurated oval patches spreading from upper extremities to lower extremities	Fevers	Eosinophils increased to 31. Biopsy of progressing rash showed dermis with dense inflammatory infiltrate consisting of numerous eosinophils and collagen bundles coated with eosinophilic granules characteristic of flame figures (Wells syndrome)	Oral corticosteroids	Improvement but patient was lost to follow-up afterwards	Friedman et al.

The intensity of associated burning pain seems to be related to subspecies in that larger centipedes, (e.g., *Scolopendra* species), inject a larger quantity of venom yielding more exaggerated symptoms [6]. Studies suggest that centipede venom activates transient receptor potential vanilloid 1 (TRPV1), which is a nociceptor that when activated transmits heat pain transduction, yielding excruciating pain [7, 22]. Cardiovascular effects, including myocardial ischemia, that have been observed in rare reports, have been associated with cardiotoxins, serotonin-like proteins and histamine components of the venom [23]. Tissue necrosis, which is commonly observed, has been associated with phospholipase A2 activity [7]. Ssm Spooky Toxin (SsTx) may also play a role in tissue necrosis as well as in vesicular cutaneous manifestations through proposed capillary vessel spasm [24]. Overall, some of the venomous components likely have a synergistic effect in the clinical manifestations observed [7].

Diagnosis

Diagnosis of centipede bite would be arduous based purely on clinical presentation and lack of history. The local reaction observed following a centipede bite can mimic cellulitis. Observation of two puncture marks at the site of fang penetration can serve as a clue and obtaining a thorough clinical history from the patient, which includes the patient's description of encountered arthropod, can guide towards an accurate diagnosis.

Treatment

Treatment for centipede bite is focused on symptom management as long as there is no superimposed bacterial infection. The affected area should be initially washed. Pain is the most common symptom associated with centipede bite and studies have demonstrated improvement in pain with ice packs and hot water immersion [25]. Oral analgesic and local lidocaine administration are other considerations for improvement of associated pain [15]. If secondary bacterial infection exists, then the underlying infection should be addressed and treated. Organisms affecting pre-existing skin lesions need to always be considered in the differential diagnosis, especially in patients with protracted course of illness and continued worsening of symptoms. For example, a case of cutaneous diphtheria, which is rare (see Table 1), has been reported following a centipede bite [26].

References

1. Undheim E, Fry B, King G. Centipede venom: recent discoveries and current state of knowledge. Toxins. 2015;7(3):679–704.
2. Bonato L, Edgecombe G, Lewis J, Minelli A, Pereira L, Shelley R, Zapparoli M. A common terminology for the external anatomy of centipedes (Chilopoda). ZooKeys. 2010;69:17–51.
3. Adis J, Harvey MS. How many Arachnida and Myriapoda are there worldwide and in Amazonia? Stud Neotropical Fauna Environ. 2000;35:139–41.
4. Minelli A, Golovatch SI. Myriapods. Encycl Biodiveres. 2013;5:421–32.
5. Edgecombe GD, Giribet G. Evolutionary biology of centipedes (Myriapoda: Chilopoda). Annu Rev Entomol. 2007;52:151–70.
6. Undheim EA, Kng GF. On the venom system of centipedes (Chilopoda), a neglected group of venomous animals. Toxicon. 2011;57:512–24.
7. Ombati R, Luo L, Yang S, Lai R. Centipede envenomation: clinical importance and the underlying molecular mechanisms. Toxicon. 2018;154:60–8.
8. Mitchell M, Tully TN. Manual of Exotic Pet Practice-E-Book. Elsevier Health Sciences; 2008. Accessed March 16, 2019.
9. Veraldi S, Chiaratti A, Sica L. Centipede bite: a case report. Arch Dermatol. 2010;146:807–8.
10. Bouchard NC, Chan GM, Hoffman RS. Vietnamese centipede envenomation. Vet Hum Toxicol. 2004;46:312–3.
11. Veraldi S, Cuka E, Gaiani F. Scolopendra bites: a report of two cases and review of the literature. Int J Dermatol. 2014;53:869e72.
12. Balit CR, Harvey MS, Waldock JM, et al. Prospective study of centipede bites in Australia. J Toxicol Clin Toxicol. 2004;42:41–8.
13. Medeiros CR, Susaki TT, Knysak I, et al. Epidemiologic and clinical survey of victims of centipede stings admitted to Hospital Vital Brazil. 2008;52:606–610.
14. Fung HT, Lam SK, Wong OF. Centipede bite victims: a review of patients presenting to two emergency departments in Hong Kong. Hong Kong Med J. 2011;17:381–5.
15. Pollack RJ, Norton SA. Ectoparasite infestations and arthropod injuries. In: Larry Jameson J et al editors. Harrison's principles of internal medicine, 20e. New York: McGraw-Hill. http://accessmedicine.mhmedical.com.online.uchc.edu/content.aspx?bookid=2129&sectionid=192534409. Accessed 26 Jan 2019.
16. Harada S, Yoshizaki Y, Natsuaki M, Shimizu H, Fukuda H, Nagai H, et al. Three cases of centipede allergy and analysis of cross reactivity with bee allergy. Jpn J Allergol. 2005;54:1279e84 (in Japanese).
17. Shimoura S, Hayashi K, Harada S, Natsuaki M. A case of centipede allergy without cross reaction to bee venom. Jpn J Dermatoallergol. 2005;13:e202 (in Japanese).
18. Washio K, Masaki T, Fujii S, Hatakeyama M, Oda Y, Fukunaga A, Natsuaki M. Anaphylaxis caused by a centipede bite: a "true" type-I allergic reaction. Allergol Int. 2018;67(3):419–20.
19. Wang IK, Hsu SP, Chi CC, Lee KF, Lin PY, Chang HW, Chuang FR. Rhabdomyolysis, acute renal failure, and multiple focal neuropathies after drinking alcohol soaked with centipede. Ren Fail. 2004;26(1):93–7.
20. Ozsarac M, Karcioglu O, Ayrik C, Somuncu F, Gumrukcu S. Acute coronary ischemia following centipede envenomation: case report and review of the literature. Wilderness Environ Med. 2004;15(2):109–12.
21. Friedman IS, Phelps RG, Baral J, et al. Wells syndrome triggered by centipede bite. Int J Dermatol. 1998;37:602–5.
22. Yang S, Yang F, Wei N, Hong J, Li B, Luo L, Rong M, Yarov-Yarovoy V, Zheng J, Wang K, Lai R. A pain-inducing centipede toxin targets the heat activation machinery of nociceptor TRPV1. Nat Commun. 2015;6:8297.

23. Yildiz A, Biçeroglu S, Yakut N, Bilir C, Akdemir RAA. Acute myocardial infarction in a young man caused by centipede sting. Emerg Med J. 2006;23:e30.
24. Luo L, Li B, Wang S, Wu F, Wang X, Liang P, Ombati R, Chen J, Lu X, Cui J, Lu Q. Centipedes subdue giant prey by blocking KCNQ channels. Proc Natl Acad Sci. 2018;115(7):1646–51.
25. Chaou CH, Chen CK, Chen JC, Chiu TF, Lin CC. Comparisons of ice packs, hot water immersion, and analgesia injection for the treatment of centipede envenomations in Taiwan. Clin Toxicol. 2009;47(7):659–62.
26. Jüngling C, Sadowski C, Glitsch M, Vandersee S. Secondary cutaneous diphtheria due to the bite of a Thai centipede (Scolopendra). JDDG: Journal der Deutschen Dermatologischen Gesellschaft. 2014;12(11):1043–4.

Index

© Springer Nature Switzerland AG 2020
J. Trevino and A.-Y. Chen (eds.), *Dermatological Manual of Outdoor Hazards*,
https://doi.org/10.1007/978-3-030-37782-3